Child Pain, Migraine, and Invisible Disability

T0187730

"The Western contemporary ethos confers innocence and nostalgia on childhood, a tendency that too often belittles, denies or oversimplifies the suffering that real children experience. Young sufferers from migraine are consummate examples of this dilemma, as Susan Honeyman documents well in *Child Pain, Migraine, and Invisible Disability*. Health care providers, who generally ask children to report pain using a reductionist single answer on a pain scale, would do well to consider Honeyman's complex, humane account (including first-person narratives)."
—*Cindy Dell Clark, Rutgers University, USA*

In the twenty-first century there is increasing global recognition of pain relief as a basic human right. However, as Susan Honeyman argues in this new take on child pain and invisible disability, such a belief has historically been driven by adult, ideological needs, whereas the needs of children in pain have traditionally been marginalized or overlooked in comparison.

Examining migraines in children and the socially disabling effects that chronic pain can have, this book uses medical, political, and cultural discourse to convey a sense of invisible disability in children with migraine and its subsequent oppression within educational and medical policy. The book is supported by authentic migraineurs' experiences and firsthand interviews as well as testimonials from a range of historical, literary, and medical sources never combined in a child-centered context before. Representations of child pain and lifespan migraine within literature, art and popular culture are also pulled together in order to provide an interdisciplinary guide to those wanting to understand migraine in children and the identity politics of disability more fully.

Child Pain, Migraine, and Invisible Disability will appeal to scholars in childhood studies, children's rights, literary and visual culture, disability studies, and medical humanities. It will also be of interest to anyone who has suffered from migraines or has cared for children affected by chronic pain.

Susan Honeyman is Professor of English at University of Nebraska at Kearney, USA.

Interdisciplinary Disability Studies
Series editor: Mark Sherry
The University of Toledo, USA

Disability studies has made great strides in exploring power and the body. This series extends the interdisciplinary dialogue between disability studies and other fields by asking how disability studies can influence a particular field. It will show how a deep engagement with disability studies changes our understanding of the following fields: sociology, literary studies, gender studies, bioethics, social work, law, education, and history. This ground-breaking series identifies both the practical and theoretical implications of such an interdisciplinary dialogue and challenges people in disability studies as well as other disciplinary fields to critically reflect on their professional praxis in terms of theory, practice, and methods.

For a full list of titles in this series, please visit www.routledge.com/series/ASHSER1401

Forthcoming:

Sport and the Female Disabled Body
Elisabet Apelmo

Disability and Rurality
Identity, Gender, and Belonging
Karen Soldatic and Kelley Johnson

Disability and Art History
Edited by Elizabeth Howie and Ann Millett-Gallant

Organizing the Blind
The Case of ONCE in Spain
Roberto Garvía

Disability and Social Media
Global Perspectives
Edited by Mike Kent and Katie Ellis

Child Pain, Migraine, and Invisible Disability

Susan Honeyman

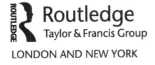

Routledge
Taylor & Francis Group

LONDON AND NEW YORK

First published 2017 by Routledge

2 Park Square, Milton Park, Abingdon, Oxfordshire OX14 4RN
52 Vanderbilt Avenue, New York, NY 10017

*Routledge is an imprint of the Taylor & Francis Group,
an informa business*

First issued in paperback 2018

British Library Cataloguing in Publication Data
A catalogue record for this book is available from the British Library

Library of Congress Cataloging in Publication Data
A catalog record for this book has been requested

ISBN: 978-1-138-20786-8 (hbk)
ISBN: 978-0-367-20819-6 (pbk)

Typeset in Times New Roman
by Apex CoVantage, LLC

For Annecy

Contents

Figures

Cover art: "*Céphalée*," by Noëla Mari by permission of the artist

Permissions

Preface

A note to readers

Imagine an unusually clever eight-year-old girl—assertive, yet soft-spoken. At this age, her attacks come about twice a week, and when they do, she has few choices. If she's at school, where she's missed so many days to migraine that her mother is frequently threatened with visits from the police, she can ask to go to the secretary's room to lie down—after 15 minutes she'll be told her permitted "rest" time is up. She is not allowed to call her mother. She can barely keep her eyes open because of the light. She won't vomit because her stomach is empty, but that doesn't make the nausea any more tolerable. When she returns to the class, still in pain, her principal comes in to denounce her in front of the other students and teacher as a liar and faker. This is a true story.

There are multiple material realities and historical forces that have led to this very point in our perverse cultural moment. Pain is the oldest of them—the bullying, probably just as old. More surprising is that migraine itself was recognized by its most distinctive features in ancient cultures. Apparently, six millennia aren't enough for humanity to learn how to treat a migraineur with adequate understanding, especially if she is a child. This is a story of child migraineurs, who are living with invisible pain and deserve more dignity and public understanding, through flexible school policies, medical research, accessible alternative therapy, and personalized coping strategies. Though young people who experience episodic or chronic impairments are sometimes thought of as *sickly* by peers and *whiny* by adults who should know better, I hope to illustrate the tough coping of *runt power*.

That child migraineurs' aura, pain, nausea, and even vomiting can nonetheless be explained away rather than believed and relieved reflects our views of children's relationships to illness, to honesty, and to their rights to determine the treatment of their bodies. In this book I will call for greater child self-determination, but also, a cutting through the thicket of webs adults create when we assume a sick child is lying.

Acknowledgments

This book is more (and at times perhaps less) than an academic project. It is the result of searching for the kind of answers and validation I yearned for during my youth in order to understand the seeming helplessness, sometimes even indifference, of adults toward the invisible pain of migraine. In this sense my book is just as much a legitimacy narrative as those I critique. To write from such a perspective (combining the personal with the professional) involved expanding my focus to include myself as one of my subjects. As my curiosity in part concerned the effects of early untreated pain on a child's future pain experiences, and my own precarious condition took place when I was too young to remember much of anything consciously, I enlisted the help of my father as co-detective, even tracking down and interviewing one of the doctors who'd been involved with my treatment. So my first thanks belong to Richard Honeyman for the fun of the search, but also for getting that second opinion so many years ago that saved my life.

I was fortunate as a child to have great medical advocates in my parents. To my mother, Mary Clemens Krehbiel Honeyman, thank you for exhausting all resources and taking a chance on alternative approaches to healing and education—without these, I can't imagine how differently my life would have turned out. Words are inadequate to express my debt of gratitude. My deepest respect and admiration goes to comrades Heidi Eichbauer, Jessica Isaac, and Shaun Friedrichsen—thank you all for your generous encouragement and insightful comments on earlier drafts. Thanks to Amanda Slater for the index, Janet Steele for translating the pathophysiology of migraine into lay terms that I could finally understand, Kurt Borchard for practical ethnographic tips, and Ralph Hanson for pushing me to "get out there and talk to people." Having the opportunity to connect with so many migraineurs in interviews was unforgettably validating and enlightening—to each of you, too many to name here, thank you for lending your voice and experience to this project; I hope this book suffices as an homage. Also a thrill was the opportunity of interviewing Dr. Joost Haan, research neurologist at the University of Leiden; pain specialist Dr. Jason Rowling; and surgeon Dr. Gil Santoscoy. Dr. Kristin Lawson and Cortney Geisler, thank you for restoring my confidence that the medical arts can be caring and healing. For inspiration and camaraderie, thanks to my classmates and instructors at the University of Leiden Law School's summer program in International Child Rights. To dear friends Marguerite Tassi and Kate Benzel, thank you for rides to get rescue meds and reminding me that one can be vulnerable with dignity.

When this book comes out I'll be close to turning 50, the age at which I'll no longer be able to take triptans for aborting attacks. It may be the beginning of an unwelcome "second childhood" for me as a migraineur. However I cope, I know that my greatest advocate and partner, William Avilés, will be there silent and still by my bedside, always pressing on my forehead just so to counter the pressure in my skull, keeping me anchored and calm. To him, my love and gratitude is a constant. It still amazes me that a loving touch really does make pain just a little bit easier to endure.

Introduction

In the last quarter of the twentieth century, discourses surrounding child health reached such a pitch and complete incompossibility that to trace current discourses back to them is both shocking and enlightening in the present. On one hand, the United States experienced an unprecedented rise in medicating children for "behavioral" conditions. On another, the medical community was becoming more conscious of a long-standing tradition of denying child vulnerability to pain, which had resulted in undermedicating neonate pain. Though antiabortion activists spread appeals based on the "silent scream" trope, they did so seemingly unaware of the fact that dominant hospital methods for circumcision, and even invasive surgeries on premature babies, were still to forego any anesthesia or analgesia as both unnecessary and risky. In contrast, pain activists like Jill Lawson promoted greater public understanding of children's pain-relief rights with a resulting call for anesthetic therapy. But the lack of a consistent public awareness about children's pain and whether to medicate their bodies betrays how readily many of those arguing did so to serve adult, ideological angles, not the actual needs of hurting children.

I am interested in teasing out the contrary logical strands in this paradoxical discursive knot, especially in the case of child migraine, which, as an episodic pain syndrome, controls out factors of contentious "cures" or fatality, allowing me to focus on how adults have historically dealt with child pain in public discourse so that I can encourage a more compassionate and effective response in our present schools, clinics, and homes. In *Child Pain, Migraine, and Invisible Disability*, I expose the historic neglect of child pain, study the dominant literary misrepresentations and lore surrounding migraine, reconstruct the bizarre material history of migraine treatments, counter stereotypes with a collection of child migraineurs' experiences, analyze children's migraine art and comics in the context of visual activism, and celebrate the everyday efforts of those who successfully cope in spite of a double bias against them as children and migraineurs, in order to show that children experiencing migraine struggle from a lack of effective treatment and from community misunderstanding, all the more complicated because their impairment is invisible, fluctuating, and silent.

The academically unexplored experience of child migraine serves as a vantage point from which to dismantle precise ableist and ageist assumptions that undergird otherwise concealed abuses of child bodies, child minds, and basic human rights:

the belief that children are less sensitive to pain, that pediatric pain is too risky to treat, that children should be quiet and relatively still (or drugged accordingly), that only women get migraine, that migraineurs are just *wimps* who complain (and so don't need treatment), or that they are *runts* who will outgrow and forget the pain (when in fact untreated child pain can create later chronic, dysfunctional pain syndromes). Against such pervasively accepted falsehoods, I will offer historical contextualization and a politicized perspective on child pain, investigate these politics within the larger history of migraine (by necessity to contrast the ubiquitous falsifying discourse representing it as an adult phenomenon), and embrace a liberatory perspective of both invisible disability and children's rights to be heard and participate in the most effective coping possible. Recognizing the oppressive power of historically unquestioned rhetoric that delegitimizes migraine and positions children as relatively immune to debilitating pain is urgent in a contemporary context in which both are met with social, medical, and educational neglect.

Decades of scholarship on disability provide multiple perspectives from which to better understand migraine experience and expressions, but migraine also complicates the rich debates to be found there, forcing a reevaluation of what constitutes resistance and agency. The hitherto untold history of *child* migraine brings to light problems for new debate within an already fascinating body of humanities scholarship on pain, uniquely urging the necessity of voicing and visual activism in particular for representing children. At the intersection of childhood studies, disability studies, and medical humanities, I find that migraine challenges intellectual efforts to idealize agency in a rejection of medicalized identity. Agency cannot simply exist in resisting medicalization, pharmaceuticals, or the mind-body dualism of the Cartesian subject. In the case of child migraine, fostering agency requires aiding young subjects in a precarious negotiation of elusive treatments, legitimacy narratives, visibility, accommodation, and solidarity forged through an understanding of neurohistory and silencing rhetoric. Much insight will be gleaned from interdisciplinary theoretical sources, but ultimately I hope to stress the embodied practices suggested by testimonies from those who actually experience migraine.

Through an analysis of medical history, literature, visual culture, and personal testimonies, my book will indicate unique complications to debates in the medical humanities and disability studies. Important developments in these subfields have fostered richly contextualized and highly nuanced work, inclusive to chronic and invisible impairments. Anne Hunsaker Hawkins indicates this trend at the beginning of the twenty-first century: "[P]athographies had undergone a kind of paradigm shift, with acute illness displaced by chronic illnesses. [P]eople were writing much more about disabilities, both major and minor—conditions that one tends neither to recover or die from. Increasingly, moreover, pathographies appeared about conditions that might not, earlier on, have been thought 'serious' enough" (124). Migraine fits this niche precisely. By integrating the methods of voicing and visibility projects, I hope to bring child migraine into "serious" public consideration. In keeping with the dictum "not for us without us," I have interviewed migraineurs and excavated testimonies from a vast and varied body of sources to piece together authentic voices on migraine, and childhood experiences in particular. However, my approach is primarily literary and political—the informal ethnographic elements making just part of a larger effort to demonstrate the pervasive rhetoric of silencing child pain and to voice possibilities for resistance.

Migraine, as an invisible impairment, would seem, like all dysfunctional pain, to defy visibility projects (visual activism), yet there is a vast body of migraine art that attempts to enable access into the experience to promote empathy and awareness in others. Within disability studies, Rosemarie Garland-Thomson has amply demonstrated that visually beholding diverse bodily forms expands our sense of the realistic human spectrum (9, 193). In *The Scar of Visibility,* Petra Kuppers considers scars as sites of cultural meaning, and like Garland-Thomson, successfully demonstrates how familiarizing images of bodily difference can neutralize stigmatization. In her chapter on migraine, Kuppers reveals an exploitative and corporately co-opting side of migraine art, further complicating visibility projects. My argument will indicate some of the hidden positives in migraine art, but more importantly it points to how differently visibility projects operate for child migraineurs, who suffer silently and stilly, only "proving" their impairment through reluctant confessions (as N. Ann Davis explains is required of persons with invisible disability in general), coerced by a suspicious mainstream norm. In this sense, children with migraine are doubly co-opted into silence by ableist *and* ageist hegemony.

Pain complicates expression, solidarity, and agency. While an upbeat atmosphere promotes "resilience" in some corners of disability studies, following the example of queer pride (exemplified by some as "crip pride"), migraineurs are unlikely to celebrate their pain as an embraceable difference or mobilize under a banner of pride, no matter how unified. So, whereas many in disability studies voice an understandable distrust of allopathic medicine and Big Pharma (criticisms which I indeed support), fighting the old fight for fair accommodations and also more aggressive treatment, even medical testing, is a necessary middle ground in the undertreated case of child migraine. Susan Wendell has explained the resulting political dilemma in the fight for recognizing chronic illnesses as socially disabled impairments: "Because disability activists have worked hard to resist medicalization and promote the social model of disability,[1] activists sometimes feel pressured to downplay the realities of fluctuating impairment or ill health," and "Outside disability activism, there is pressure to conform to an inspiring version of the paradigm of disability" (22). Alison Kafer writes that

> the social model with its impairment/disability distinction erases the lived realities of impairment; in its well-intentioned focus on the disabling effects of society, it overlooks the often-disabling effects of our bodies. People with chronic illness, pain, and fatigue have been among the most critical of this aspect of the social model, rightly noting that social and structural changes will do little to make one's joints stop aching or to alleviate back pain.

(7)

Any study of migraine requires not just a focus on how to accommodate those impaired, but also to understand where medical intervention, no matter how flawed, is necessary. As a "fluctuating impairment," migraine allows migraineurs to pass on good days as unimpaired, thus complicating needs for accommodation on bad days—either way, eluding the liberatory paradigm of disability in such a way that requires a balance between calls for social justice *and* advocating for better treatment. While critiquing oppressive social factors (such as adult exploitation of child controllability) and voicing resilience, I hope to pragmatically impress upon my readers the therapeutic importance of negotiating medical interventions with critical awareness. *Child Pain, Migraine, and Invisible Disability* combines a social history of child pain, material/literary analysis of migraine, and a diverse set of intimate perspectives in order to ultimately foster an informed sense of community among child migraineurs through shared politics and their own bodily resources of healing, or "runt power."

Language and literary disciplines contribute to disability nuance through subtle discourse and phenomenological analysis. Mark Sherry indicates that the performative/constructivist trend in literary scholarship in recent decades "helps us to understand that disability and impairment are both social constructs. This is important, because a great deal of disability studies tends to assume that impairment is simply a biological given, which is inscribed on the body" (2005, 167). Though I will often fall back on the impairment (biological) versus disability (social) paradigm for expediency and where necessary for simple clarity, Sherry's point that both are ultimately discursively inflected categories helps to suggest the importance of interdisciplinary work on disability and impairment as concepts in the constant negotiation of identity at the intersection of individual experiences and social forces that confine yet set the stage for such "performances." As social constructs both the medical and social aspects of migraine are subject to discursive interpretations, at which the humanities excel. Whereas my project will lack the rigorous scientific design and controls of medical study, sociological/anthropological ethnography, or psychology, I hope its value can be found in providing critical contextualization for propelling conversation, beyond doctors' offices and patients' blogs, about the cultural meanings of migraine and phenomenological experiences of migraineurs, encouraging greater understanding of a fairly underrepresented contingent of that group, children, who need to be included in the conversation. Toward this end my book necessarily focuses more broadly on pain and migraine throughout social history and the individual lifespan. And in order to begin answering why it has remained so culturally dismissed, I need to consider migraine in the larger history of child pain. To come nearer to understanding what child migraineurs share with migraineurs of all ages, I draw where relevant from knowledge about the latter as well (often relying on the retrospective testimony of adults with migraine who also experienced the attacks in childhood). This allows me to draw important contrasts into sharper definition, indicating areas of experience unique to child migraineurs.

This book is also unapologetically personal, as I myself was a child migraineur, so rather than fronting an impossible and disingenuous "objectivity," I take the liberty of reserving a brief afterword for my own personal testimony about migraine to add to the chorus. The personal is, after all, political, and in the case of invisible disability, I believe concrete examples from the everyday lives of ordinary people can be helpful in demonstrating how deeply the hegemony of ableism extends, how it uniquely affects children, and also how it can be individually (and thus collectively) resisted.

Intersecting with the child-rights rhetoric that infuses my previous work in childhood studies, the following chapters should expose the silencing discourses of power that operate in the politics of pediatric pain and literary migraine, counter that silence by voicing undertreated perspectives of migraine experience, and demonstrate multiple efforts to legitimize migraine by focusing on material realities (which I will argue constitutes visual activism but can also trivialize through romanticization and essentializing). I hope to advocate a unified awareness of our bodily vulnerabilities for everyone (which Ruth O'Brien calls "animality"), using the subject of child migraine as an anchoring case to visualize and empathize with the pain of others, encouraging a coping culture. Those interested in childhood studies and child rights will find new evidence and deeper historical contextualization for understanding how child pain has been silenced and how we might foster voicing the muted perspectives of children in pain. For readers interested in the medical humanities, I hope to indicate the relevance of childhood studies to bioethics and demonstrate the risks of metaphor in promoting empathy, which in turn complicate the voicing projects of childhood studies. In these efforts, much can be learned from the solidarity and visual activism of disability politics. And in a mutually productive manner, consideration of migraine in the context of disability studies further complicates the possibilities there for envisioning agency that can negotiate the precarious ideologies and identity politics involved in resisting allopathic healing as medicalizing, simply co-opted by the pharmaceutical industry, or psychologically stereotyped out of individual recognition. Listening to multiple individual perspectives in this new context is just the beginning of understanding child pain and coping as a personally embodied *and* socially shared experience.

There are no books that I am aware of, within the humanities, which address child migraine as the sole subject. Even within medical subfields, the only large-scale, book-length, and comprehensively focused study of child migraine is Bo Bille's from 1962. Migraine is most commonly thought of as an adult problem, which is a damaging misconception. In fact 10% of children will experience some degree of migraine disability during their childhood, and about 6% of any given population (about half of all migraineurs) will get their first attack before age 12. There is great need for more interdisciplinary scholarship on the challenges of migraine experience that are unique to children. Unfortunately, most books for nonmedical readers on migraine are limited to the self-help genre, but there are also several delightful migraine and chronic-headache memoirs, like Andrew Levy's *A Brain Wider Than the Sky*, Jennette Fulda's *Chocolate and Vicodin*, and Paula Kamen's *All in My Head*. The first widely read text for a general audience on the subject was *Migraine*, by Oliver Sacks, which has never been out of print since 1970. The success of *Migraine*, headache memoirs, and sophisticated journalistic works like Melanie Thernstrom's *The Pain Chronicles* indicates a demand for the thinker's alternative to *Mommy, My Head Hurts*.

This book is organized into five chapters, a conclusion, and afterword with a cumulatively personal tone, first balancing empirical with subjective perspectives to ultimately blend social and phenomenological views of child migraine to utilize strengths of each approach. Following a case for understanding (child) migraine as a disability in chapter 1, I will begin to dig deeper into history to explain why it has been overlooked. In chapter 2, "A History of Pediatric Pain and the Politics of Pill Culture," I demonstrate the history of denying, and sometimes taking advantage of, child pain in order to contextualize our present paradox of undertreating child pain but overmedicating inconvenient child behaviors. This context will be crucial to understanding how impairments like migraine have been uniquely socially disabling for children through lack of proper understanding or accommodation. Understanding the role of institutions in the social disability of migraineurs as therapeutic orphans in zero-tolerance, assessment-focused schools requires exposing the hypocrisy of adult-serving ideologies (that can, whether intentionally or not, exploit the controllability of children). Playing on the name of the troublesome trigeminal nervous system crucial in triggering migraine attacks, I will call the ideologies of silencing child pain, as well as the (sometimes literally) paralyzing control of migraine, "trigemony." As if in collusion with the hegemonic forces of educational and medical policies, the attacks subdue the child migraineur. By unsilencing child pain we can more clearly recognize socially disabling features of childhood institutions.

To flesh out my depiction of institutional restrictions from chapters 1 and 2, the next half of the book will trace literary stereotypes and compensatory narratives countered with phenomenological perspectives afforded by authentic individual experiences, filling in gaps from the medical and social models of disease and disability. In chapter 3, "Materia Medica," I consider how a revolt against trigemony can be violent, but also how pain has been reduced to mere metaphor in the public imagination, and migraine has been trivialized. The resulting "legitimacy deficit" (Joanna Kempner) demands concretized corrective evidence, attempted in "materializing" processes (Justine S. Murison), from literature and illustration to neuroimaging, that represent this invisible impairment for others to imagine. To set up my own analysis of materializing practices (of confessional narratives in chapter 4 or migraine art and comics in chapter 5), I here trace misrepresentations that usually center on stereotypes (especially the idle, wealthy, white mother figure) and subtler compensatory narratives that reveal and reinforce misleading profiles of migraine that contribute to keeping child migraineurs culturally invisible.

Literary representations of migraine are preoccupied with negotiating the tensions between trivialization and legitimization. A popular legitimizing method (that also can contribute to trivialization) can be seen in critics' tendency toward posthumously "diagnosing" artists and authors as migraineurs—projecting migraine onto already-legitimated subjects. The most famous example of this process can be seen in readings of Lewis Carroll (after whom a migraine aura, "Alice in Wonderland syndrome," is even named). Ultimately, such compensatory outings reveal a lot about where and how atypical neurological experience is revered, and why it is not elsewhere. Literary expressions that celebrate visual aura of migraineurs tend to downplay the more troublesome issue of pain, the more universal (and usually more debilitating) symptom. Some even romanticize migraine aura, and the tendency is to focus entirely on *visual* aura, even though migraine (like epileptic) aurae can affect any of the senses and mobility, and even encompass emotional states. The erasure of migraine pain in literary figurations, like the denial of child pain in medical history, depletes empathy and increases the invisibility of child migraineurs in popular discourse.

Woven into my analysis of migraine representations is a contextualizing material history of treatments, which have always played a role in the personal cost-benefit analysis of pain relief. Though focused on the material body, my goal in this chapter is to make more explicit the discursive positioning of migraineurs, through various "cure" theories and marginalizing definitions echoing the deeper riff from chapter 2, a pervasive reluctance to recognize and treat child pain. The relationships between a migraineur's body and the social world cover a range of interventions, including trepanation, folk remedies, quackery, opiates/opioids, cannabis, ergot, anticonvulsants and infusions, supplements, and what is sometimes called the "triptan revolution"; these have generally excluded prepubescent migraineurs, a dilemma which I will contextualize within the "therapeutic orphan" issue of undertreating children due to undertesting (a thorny child-rights issue). In contrast, I will briefly look at alternative methods historically constructed as kid friendly, such as elimination diets (food allergy), acupuncture, biofeedback, distraction, and guided imagery. Children are particularly skillful in utilizing alternative methods to allopathic healing, and in this sense I will celebrate their unique potential for coping.

Pain is a controversial, ineffable phenomenon (Elaine Scarry), and its invisibility unfortunately makes it possible to attribute pain to those who are not in pain, falsely justifying the abuse of nonverbally impaired persons (Siebers 2010). But it also allows for the cultural erasure of real pain in marginalized persons. One of the challenges of representing invisible impairments is to voice the pain of others without patheticizing (I use the term "migraineur" instead of the diplomatically favored "person with migraine," unfortunately ubiquitous "migraine sufferer," or patronizing "victim of migraine"). The best way to do this, we learn from the ethnographic work of Myra Bluebond-Langner and Cindy Dell Clark, is by relying heavily on their own words. So in chapter 4, "Testifying against Trigemony," I weave a collection of migraineurs' experiences (based on original interviews[2] and eclectic anecdotes). Testimonies suggest that the current popularity of transcending mind-body dualism in favor of integrated, embodied identity is not so consistently applicable in the case of migraine, which, like many pain conditions, requires "out-of-body" distraction (albeit imaginary) as a coping strategy.

Susan Wendell theorizes the importance of recognizing individual experiences of chronic illness as a means of recognizing difference, rectifying social disability of that difference, yet doing so without silencing or increasing suffering: "The perspectives of people with chronic illnesses will be essential to such an exploration, because it may be as difficult for healthy disabled people to see the value of illness as for nondisabled people to see the value of disability" (31). Testimonies will help me to illustrate individual experiences, along with excerpts from migraine diaries that articulate invisible disability experienced in childhood and adolescence—especially the vague impression that others think one is weak or essentially *sickly* to be so affected by "just a headache." I use the term "runt" to convey the resulting internalized sense of puniness and the impression of being "cast out" of the healthy, or thriving, community, but I also hope it conveys that baldly confronting the vulnerability of our animal bodies invites solidarity and strength through compassionate interdependence.

Taking my next chapter title, "Visibility Machines and Pain Proxies," in part from the work of Petra Kuppers, I analyze migraine art, children's books, and comics in the context of the demarginalizing politics of disability studies. In the explosive example of Friedrich Nietzsche, the somber expression of Reneé French, and the levity of George Herriman, I celebrate affirming projections in the effort to resist migraine and fortify the self. These migraineurs have modeled the coping power of projecting pain onto an imaginary proxy, thereby providing a textual enactment of the coping technique called imaging, a technique at which children in particular excel.

I am aware of the exploitative potential of an adult trying to represent the political interests of children, especially where it concerns something as intimate and disempowering as pain. Child-rights icon Janusz Korczak wrote, in his *Ghetto Diary*, that "[t]o describe someone else's pain resembles thieving, preying upon misfortune, as if there were not enough of it as things are" (40–41). As a result, I feel it is politically necessary (and strikingly precedented within disability studies[3]) to foreground my subjective investment in this study by including my own testimony about experiencing migraine as a child, and in telling contrast, as an adult. In a brief afterword, "Scars," my own migraine diary demonstrates an embodied example of migraine experience, illustrating some of the unique challenges of child migraine and my larger argument in a more personalized tenor. Here I hope to translate the more complicated possibilities for agency in one individual's concrete (albeit idiosyncratic) experience, demonstrating that migraineurs can feel solidarity through shared experience, but also self-affirmation in the acknowledgment *and* rejection of pain. We might be migraineurs, but we are *not* migraine.

Notes

1 Rachel Adams makes the social model of disability vividly accessible in this explanation: "Rather than fixating on illness or impairment, they [scholars and activists] were concerned with the environmental factors that excluded full participation in the social world. A person in a wheelchair was disabled by stairs and broken elevators, not by her inability to walk" (196).

2 Negotiating the limitations of my own discipline with recognition of the necessity in disability politics for self-representation ("not for us without us"), I've collected informal ethnographic evidence through word-of-mouth referrals that led to one- to three-hour recorded interviews with 30 migraineurs who were given the choice to be anonymous, go

by a chosen alias, or be identified by name. When impossible otherwise, due to distance, I carried out two of these interviews via phone and one via email. The questionnaire I followed can be found in the appendix at the end of the book, but I learned much more from the conversations that naturally digressed. I also benefited from interviewing a migraine artist, one pain specialist, a neurologist researcher, and a surgeon who worked with pediatric cases in the seventies, which he called "a very bad time for children in medicine."

3   Most relevant to my overall method are the rhetorical models to be seen in Mark Sherry's *If I Only Had a Brain: Deconstructing Brain Injury* (2006), Stuart Murray's *Representing Autism: Culture, Narrative, Fascination* (2008), Margaret Price's *Mad at School: Rhetorics of Mental Disability and Academic Life* (2011), and Jenny Slater's *Youth and Disability: A Challenge to Mr. Reasonable* (2015). These works demonstrate interdisciplinary methods and source work, as well as honestly presenting the author's subjective investment as an asset to directly demonstrating embodied experience. I agree with Murray's recognition that "the *only* way to write, comment and analyse is to work from such a position of partiality. . . . The readings are personal, as the book is as a whole, but that does not, I would assert, mean it cannot be scholarly" (18–19). Like Price and Slater, I also utilize interviews not as scientific data but to democratize my rhetorical approach. Susannah B. Mintz argues that pain, in particular, "reduces everything to itself, dominating consciousness in a way that seems to collapse identity into the maddening persistence of discomfort," making it a perceptual experience that "needs to be examined within the context of a person's whole familial, social, psychological, emotional, corporeal history" (2011, 243–245). She views "the lyric essay as pain's most suitable autobiographical genre" (245).

1 Migraine as invisible disability

"The difference between a headache and a migraine is like the difference between being tapped by a push pin and stabbed by a machete."

Nathan Speer

"It feels really hot, like a tool banging in my head, gashing into my head with a hammer."

Annecy Crockett

It begins with a blip in the electrical impulses of the nervous system. Cerebral blood flow goes haywire providing phantom sensory experiences that signal the worst is coming—a pain that for some is excruciating. The nerves go haywire, too—especially the trigeminal branch so close to our sensory inputs (nose, ears, and especially the eyes, around which the pain throbs and radiates). These symptoms distract us from the gut, which like a tangled garden hose might lie kinked for days—it seems lifeless except for the waves of nausea and occasional vomiting (Fields 176). This set of symptoms harkens us to retreat into silence, stillness, and dark. But when you are little and something scares you, you run and hide or call to others for help. Something hurts—you will pull a face, cry, or distract yourself in play. All of these quite reasonable reactions make a migraine attack even worse.

Migraine has existed and been recognized, at least by its most notable symptoms (moderate to severe unilateral head pain, nausea/vomiting, photophobia and phonophobia, and for many, a range of prodromal aurae including hallucination, partial blindness, or paralysis), as long as history has been written.[1] It has existed for so long that, at least in the English lexicon, it has become an overused term that the general public simply confuses for a "bad headache," much to the chagrin of migraineurs. Though culturally misunderstood, it has long been recognized in healing professions as both widespread and potentially debilitating. Edgar A. Hines wrote in 1938 that "headache is probably the most universal disability afflicting mankind" and migraine "undoubtedly heads up the list of disabling headaches" (988). But migraine is not simply a headache. The World Health Organization now considers migraine as debilitating as dementia, acute psychosis, and quadriplegia and chronic migraine as disabling as rheumatoid arthritis, paraplegia, or blindness[2]

(Harwood et al. 2004). One "group of investigators estimated that migraineurs in the U.S. spend more than three million days in bed each month. . . . Each year the condition costs the U.S. approximately $1.4 billion in lost work productivity" (Lerner et al. 699). Migraine is relatively common; high estimates say that 1 in every 7, low estimates 1 in 10, adults will experience at least one migraine attack in their lifetime, whereas "3–7% of the pediatric population suffer from migraine" (Hernandez-Latorre and Roig 573). For many the condition is not too debilitating and simply episodic, but those severely, frequently, and chronically affected are generally seen as "disabled" by it: "The most disabled half of patients with migraine, for instance, account roughly for 90% of lost work time attributable to migraine" (Loder and Biondi 136). The functionalist bias of such measurements and rankings obscures the diversity of impaired experience in its reduction to numbers. By focusing on labor productivity in the case of migraine, entities like the World Health Organization overlook an entire contingent of the population that is implicitly not worth consideration.

What's ignored in most stats-loving studies is that migraine impairs kids, too. A surprising majority of the numerous publications on migraine ignore child migraineurs completely, some rife with exclusionary logic that renders them inaccurate as a result of the oversight. But it could be argued that, like asthma and other conditions that often disproportionately affect children, who sometimes luckily outgrow them, migraine should be of particular interest to generalist pediatricians, school nurses, and disability advocates, not just specialists in pediatric neurology. This isn't new news. Edward Liveing wrote in 1873 that "[m]ost of the writers on megrim and sick-headache have observed how frequently the malady makes its first appearance in childhood, and how seldom it commences after the age of thirty," adding that his eighteenth-century predecessor, Samuel-Auguste Tissot, claimed "that cases often begin at the age of seven and eight (period of second dentitions), and even much earlier" (23).

Many think of migraines exclusively as an adult, or a woman's, problem, but before puberty, slightly more males than females get them.[3] And in the more limited literature focusing specifically on child migraine, it is still widely agreed that among adult migraineurs, many first experienced attacks in their youth. According to Laura Slap-Shelton, "Approximately half of all people with migraines have had their first one by the age of 20 years" (354). The Migraine Research Foundation estimates younger, with half of migraines starting by age 12. According to Hernandez-Lorre and Roig, children with a family history of migraine are more likely to start showing symptoms before the age of 10" (575). Slap-Shelton reports "an increase in prevalence at around the age of 7 years" (354). In my own interviews with migraineurs, I was surprised to hear how many, like me, recalled "the fourth grade," in particular, as a rite of passage in pain. The fact that I so often heard "my fourth grade year" rather than "when I was 9 or 10 years old" is, in retrospect I now see, significant. Our expression of such an intimate bodily experience is nonetheless inflected by institutional frames of reference, indicating awareness of disability as a social, not simply health, issue. Whether consciously or not these migraineurs were counting back their memories in the school of pain.

More than one study suggests that headache is among the most common reasons for leaving school ill (Kuttner 286). Francis J. DiMario Jr. surveyed nurses at 256 Connecticut schools, who ranked childhood headache "behind minor trauma, GI upset, and URI as the fourth of the 13 most common clinical problems encountered at school" (279). Winner and Rothner report that "[t]he National Health Interview Survey revealed that the headache ranks third among illness-related causes of school absence" (136). It might not come as a great surprise, then, that among child migraineurs, the top factor reported as triggering and aggravating attacks is "school stress" (Passachier and Orlebeke 167). For many, the attacks first present at the beginning of schooling. Matti Sillanpää and Pirjo Anttila found that "[a]t preschool age, disturbing headache is rare, occurring in 4% to 20% of children in population studies. At school entry, markedly higher prevalences of headache have been reported, ranging from 38% to 50%" (1996, 466). Note, this statistic is for headache in general (thus the high number), including but not specific to migraine, but it speaks to stress as an aggravating factor and the telling timing of such stressors. In another study Sillanpää noted that "[h]eadache increases clearly in prevalence during the early school years. The sharpest rise occurred in the frequency category '1–4 attacks a month'" (1983, 18). D. W. Lewis et al. found that for migraine in particular, "the only causes children rated more highly than school, exercise, tension, pressure, and worry were sunglare, bright light, and loud noise, as sensitivity to which, of course, is a symptom of their actual condition" (225). I also noted in my interviews that younger subjects were more likely to report symptoms of prodrome or attack as triggers, whereas older subjects recognized that the painful perceptions of light as blinding, smells as stronger, and sounds as unbearably loud actually reflects their own hypersensitivity within the migrainous state, thus more clearly separating external and internal phenomena.

Frequency and severity of migraine become worse around school exams. In his landmark study of child migraineurs, Bo Bille found that "[a] migraine attack often occurs before, during, or after important school examinations" (1962, 21). He stresses, "*In more than half of all the children the attacks begin in connection with schoolwork, and then most often* after *schooltime*" (1962, 60). Bener et al. found that "there was a strong relationship between migraine and the timing of examinations" as well as periods of heavy homework (152, 155). Studies consistently show this connection regardless of culture: Bille's studies were of Swedish children, Sillanpää's of Finnish children, Bener's of children in the United Arab Emirates (the other studies presented here surveyed North Americans). Bener et al. nonetheless qualify a key commonality in their disclaimer:

> In [UAE] culture, academic achievement by children is an extremely pertinent issue. Often emphasis is on achieving high grades in examinations at the expense of enjoyable learning. Children are often subjected to these stresses, and complaints of headache are common, particularly during the examination season.
>
> (524)

American studies confirm these pressures as primary factors in the United States as well: "Fear of failure and school problems, but not achievement motivation, had significant positive correlations with headache complaints after correction for differences in sex and age" (Passchier and Orlebeke 167). Winner and Rothner report that "[a]lmost 2 out of 5 children with migraine (37%) report that they perform poorly during headache" (136). Liisa Metsähonkala adds that "[t]he association of stress in school with headache was strongest in girls with migraine, even though they reported the least difficulties in school subjects" (222). The stress of testing and concurrent anxieties about testing are both high and unnecessary. In contrast, "Many school children are completely free from attacks during the holidays,[4] and not infrequently children become free of symptoms when they change their teacher or their class, or leave the school" (Bille 1967, 24).

Some believe that incidence (number of attacks) and prevalence (number of persons diagnosed) for migraine have been increasing over the past 30 years. Stang et al. found that in one county of Minnesota, "From 1979 to 1981, there was a striking increase in the age-adjusted incidence of those under 45 years of age: the incidence increased 34% in women and 100% for men" (1657). Though they note an increase "across all ages," unfortunately U.S. studies on this issue tend to exclude the youngest migraineurs from their count, but Stang et al. did find their highest increase among the youngest group they tallied, 10- to 14-year-olds, not surprisingly the ages following the fourth-grade crisis period in which tracking and heaviest testing have begun. T. D. Rozen et al. found that from roughly 1979 to 1990 the number of new diagnoses of migraine among all ages increased, 88.8% in females and 39.7% in males under nine years of age (1468–70). Ishaq Abu-Arefeh and George Russell write that "[s]tudies from the United States showed a significant increase in the prevalence of chronic migraine from 25.8% to 41% between 1980 to 1989 in the adult population, but no comparable paediatric data are available" (765). Joanna Bourke reports that "[i]n 2011 and 2012, between 6 and 24 percent of people in North America and 15 percent of Europeans suffered from migraine," which she holds as "evidence of epidemic-level distress" (24). But again, the studies she cites do not indicate a consistent measure of children affected.

Fortunately, however, Finnish researchers were paying much attention to the issue in children during the same time period. Matti Sillanpää and teams surveyed Finnish schoolchildren in 1974, 1992, and 2002 maintaining the exact schools, method, and questions asked, finding that "[i]n 1974, a grossly linear increase was seen in the prevalence of migraine with age, but in 1992 the curve appeared substantially steeper from the age of 5 years," clearly indicating school as a primary stressor (1996, 469). The increases they found were shocking. For example, the increase of childhood headache in general (including nonmigrainous) went "from 14.4% in 1974 to 51.5% in 1992" (1996, 466). During the same time period, "the prevalence of migraine headache had increased from 1.9% to 5.7%" (468). These results may be inflated slightly due to the broader, older definition of migraine (Vahlquist's) they maintained in order to keep their criteria consistent, even though more current definitions[5] have narrowed. Antilla explains, "If we had chosen the

ICHD-II criteria in 1974, 1992, and 2002, the incidence rates might be slightly lower, but an increasing trend in the incidence of migraine would be apparent" (2006, e1199). These studies at the very least suggest that more research should be done to consider the factors of social environment: "The increase cannot be ascribed to the changes in the physical school environments, which have been astonishingly stable.[6] . . . [C]hanges in the social environment might explain the significantly increased prevalence. That is an alarming sign of the stressful life and ill-being of children. It may reflect the ill-being of society" (Sillanpää and Anttila 1996, 470). I would like to be able to say that a primary ill in this case is authoritarian classrooms and heavy testing, but the Finnish educational experience in no way parallels that in the United States during the time period in question. In fact, it is practically the inverse of the American trend of heavy testing (Darling-Hammond 167). Since the 1970s, Finnish schools have reformed toward no standardized testing with great success, by 2006 leading the world as a model school system. It is possible, though, that these reforms are part of a child-focused climate that would lead researchers to actually pay attention to child issues like migraine and its institutional stressors. It will be significant, indeed, to see if Finnish researchers have seen any improvement in child migraine following the actual achievement of the aimed-for success of its education reforms.

In the United States, concurrent with the rise of heavy testing and zero-tolerance policies, there has also been a slow decline in the number of nurses assigned to care for students in school, to the point that nurses often serve many schools or entire districts, rotating between them rather than serving as a health-care contact who is available during all school hours for students who have urgent but unpredictable needs. Karen Ray Stratford reports, in her 2013 Nursing thesis, that "[t]he National Association of School Nurses (NASN) recommends a nurse-to-student ratio of 1 nurse to every 750 regular education students. Most states fall far below this recommendation with the average school nurse servicing at least two schools and over 1151 students" (3). This arrangement leads to rotations wherein a student might only have a nurse in the school to turn to on one or two days of the week—not sufficient care for fluctuating, contagious, or urgent conditions. Such cutbacks will clearly leave schools even less capable of dealing with chronic conditions, like migraine, on the rise.

In the meantime, several valid speculations as to contributing factors in the increase of child migraine have been suggested. Among them, a "general trend of decreasing sleep," "increase in use of information technology," and, as Billie Joe Armstrong would sing, "soda pop" (Anttila 2006, e1200). Anttila et al. explain, "Soft-drink consumption more than doubled among children and adolescents aged 6–17 years between 1977–1978 and 1994–1998. At the same time, we found more than double the risk of migraine or frequent headache among 7-year old children in 2002 compared with 1974. Increased use of soft drinks may be related to recurrent headaches in children" (e1201). Unfortunately, the only related American study I could find that explicitly considered soft drinks in the acknowledgment that "[d]iet, stress . . . may precipitate migraine attacks" also excluded children from the study with the erroneous and marginalizing logic, "Subjects less than 12 years old . . . were excluded from the analysis because of concerns regarding ability to respond to and interpret questions" (Stewart et al. 65). But there has been targeted consideration of Anttila's speculation, at least, in a study of the correlation between caffeine and general headache in the United States, finding "approximately 55% of caffeine intake in young American schoolchildren is in the form of soft drinks" (Hering-Hanit and Gadoth, 334). Hering-Hanit and Gadoth recorded 36 patients, aged 6–18, over a five-year period, whom they persuaded to "discontinue daily use of cola drinks" (333). They concluded,

> This led to a complete cessation of all headaches in 33 out of the 36 subjects at the end of 2 weeks following cola drinks discontinuation. . . . In one boy and two adolescent girls, the daily headache was replaced by intermittent episodic migraine without aura not frequent enough to justify migraine prophylaxis.
> (333–334)

Lumping migraine with nonmigrainous headaches in this study is a bit misleading. Only seven of the children in the study had a family history of migraine, so it is much more likely that the nonmigrainous headaches were eliminated with reduction of caffeine, but only half or fewer of the migraines were.

Migraineurs have a complicated relationship with caffeine, which is both a possible trigger for attacks and aid to aborting them. Caffeine is even an ingredient in some abortive migraine medications, including being the only additive to Excedrin's standard dosage of aspirin and acetaminophen to make it Excedrin Migraine. In fact, according to one source, the caffeinated syrup for Coca-Cola was invented "as a remedy for 'sick headache'" (Sheftell 1997, 191). In the case of soda and migraines, an even more likely culprit is the sugar, which has been far more ubiquitous in the American diet and worthy of serious attention. Often overlooked in more recent literature on the disease (except where lost among the enormous list of possible dietary triggers we are warned against), sugar was understood early on by doctors as a problem for many migraineurs. In 1923, G. R. Minot went as far as to suggest that migraineurs have "some congenital or acquired defect in the carbohydrate metabolism. . . . Quite often the patient will recall that paroxysms follow the excessive intake of candy or other form of carbohydrate" (719–20). G. N. W. Thomas would advise in 1924 that "many persons who now regularly suffer from migraine will find the attacks disappear entirely if sugar be eliminated from the diet" (598). In 1949, C. F. Wilkinson Jr. confirmed that erratic glucose levels were prevalent in migraineurs, and that many could be helped with "low carbohydrate and, or, high protein diets as being of benefit in migraine" (209). Rodolfo Low promises in his 1987 book *Victory over Migraine* that by reducing intake of sucrose and stabilizing hypoglycemia, migraineurs can reduce their attacks. Low describes one patient, Anna, whose migraine attacks began at age 14, causing her to miss many school days and leading doctors to prescribe her "a variety of tranquilizers over the years on a regular basis" (4). When asked, at her first appointment, what she'd eaten that day, Anna reported, "Oh, nothing at all really. Just a Coke and a piece of cake" (5). And so runs a familiar story in migraine circles—the doctor prescribed a low-sucrose diet, and "in eighteen years Anna has not had one attack" (5). Changes in dietary lifestyle can clearly affect the increase in migraine incidence and prevalence, indicating larger cultural shifts in the food industry as aggravating factors.

Certainly the increasingly perilous standard American diet[7] is implicated as one of many possible factors. One of the first tasks toward management most migraine patients are required to do is a headache diary documenting daily pain and their arduous, protracted diagnostic isolation of food triggers through an elimination diet. But there are so many potential triggers hidden in ubiquitous processed food that finding them can take years, even decades, and avoiding them is costly. Recent research suggests that even more invisibly, the individual microbiomes of our digestive systems play a key role as well (Gershon 1998, Fields 2009, Enders 2015). For those of us with medically precarious childhoods, early antibiotic use may be a culprit, interfering with the necessary development of digestive bacteria as part of our immunity, neurotransmitter balance, and metabolism. In fact, the peripheral autonomic nervous system of our gut, called the enteric nervous system, may have an even more determinant role, and has come to be called the "second brain." Migraineurs often have high levels of glutamate (which regulates excitation, including pain signals) and low levels of serotonin (which helps stop these signals). These are manufactured in the gut. In fact, 95% of the body's serotonin is produced there (Gershon xii). If we can create the proper environment in our digestive systems to support the right bacteria to flourish, we might be able to repair this imbalance. Amongst multiple fads (some more legitimate[8] than others), one recommends choosing vegetable fats rather than animal fats, as well as taking diversifying probiotics in an effort to boost the gut's production of serotonin (Enders 47, 54–55, 138–139). One of the many reasons opioids are not advisable for migraine except in extreme, acute circumstances is that they also interfere with serotonin production, thus ultimately escalating the problem in the longer-term context. They are usually inadequate and provide only fleeting relief anyway, and are likely to trigger rebound headaches, so are only used for unusually severe or interminable attacks.

Another possibility for an apparent increase in diagnosis is simply that child migraine has become more recognized by the public and so more reported—Judith Warner points out that the perceived "autism 'epidemic' provides a very good example of how a disorder's becoming visible can lead to the perception that it has become more common" (49). If this affect also applies in the case of child migraine, the condition still needs to become more understood. Our categorizations can become overwhelmingly simplified in popular discourse. Greater visibility needs to come with a nuanced understanding of individualized suffering and how it is compounded by our institutions and the ideologies that sustain them. Michael Taussig explains that "disease is recruited into serving the ideological needs of the social order, to the detriment of healing and our understanding of the social causes of misfortune" (3). If migraine is truly experienced and/or diagnosed more frequently, what does that say about the social environment potential young migraineurs inhabit? We need to give child migraine greater consideration within the context of the history of educational institutions in the era of globalization and service economies, in which particular triggers are out of control. Maggie Jones writes, in *Your Child: Headaches and Migraine*, that "[p]ressures at school to achieve are more severe than they have ever been, with traditional manual jobs disappearing and more and more careers dependent on educational qualifications, and more and more competition[9] for jobs" (94). And with these pressures come expectations that students should passively adapt. Toby Miller argues that the result could be

> viewed as preparation for a conservative role in the labor pool, via the suppression of disgruntled responses to oppressive institutions and norms, and the diversion of energy into recreational pastimes rather than politics. A . . . more polite population reduces the cost of public health and guarantees a functioning and pliable workforce.
>
> (147)

Perhaps if we recognize the larger motivations behind our privileging the control of children over listening to their needs, we might foster healthier development.

The extent to which socioeconomic structures underlie normatizing thought about dis/ability is usually transparent: most journalistic pieces on migraine for a general audience measure disability by citing how many hours are lost to it in terms of labor productivity, and even more often these lost hours are translated into a dollar amount. Margaret H. Vickers explains that "[i]n a capitalist, functionalist society, any level of illness that takes the person below optimal capacity becomes a problem" (197). We too easily take functionality for granted as a standard even when it rigidly entraps rather than helps children. In contrast, scholars and activists in disability politics invite acknowledgment of "crip time." Alison Kafer writes that

> [c]rip time is flex time not just expanded and exploded; it requires reimagining our notions of what can and should happen in time, or recognizing how expectations of 'how long things take' are based on very particular minds and bodies.
>
> (27)

In order to realize flex time, we have to decenter functionalist time as seen through impaired perspectives. Ashley Meunchen, a Detroit-based fibers artist and migraineur since childhood, translated her own experience into an almost mock-Tayloresque parody of functionalist time in her student-exhibit piece entitled "Headache Diary." Though Meunchen usually is an abstract artist, her migraines became so uncontrollable during her final year in college that she decided to make her own headache diary more public. Mounted together are 21 small needlepoints representing the attacks she had from December 2014 to March 2015, showing milligrams of meds taken, hours and minutes counting duration, as well as pain rated on a pain scale between 1 and 10. Some exhibit visitors actually pulled out their phones to calculate the totals for her "sick time" out of the school studio to grasp a perspective of migraine time. But "Headache Diary" also renders the measures we rely upon to make our impairment real to others meaningless. The colors are intentionally as drab as numbers are. Meunchen explains, "I wanted it to be like something you'd expect to see on your grandmother's wall" (interview). The reduction of four migrainous months to a series of numbers also echoes her exasperated humor. As Vickers has stated, functional time is an assumption of capitalism "in which health is a commodity and responsibility for illness is increasingly seen to be the individual's responsibility" (197). Meunchen's exhibit challenges these assumptions, perhaps most explicitly in her needlepoint repeating "I will not get a migraine" a dozen times, usually in dull yellow, but with one central line in red. The title of the piece is "Useless Mantra."

Mel Y. Chen[10] provides another depiction of flex time as experienced with migraine in discussing "a miserable six weeks of ongoing migraines and nausea, accompanied by wiggy visual and auditory distortions," in which

> there was exactly one two-day stretch in which I was free of major head pain. I had to email excuses in advance, when I was able to read a screen and not throw up at the same time, or retrospectively apologize if I had not been able. Even harder was that it seemed extremely difficult to think, both before and after the migraine itself.
>
> (2014)

The "brain fog" and "nausea" encroach on "functionality" in ableist time as well as the pain, adding yet another dimension of alterity. Michelle Martinovic, whose migraine attacks began when she was five years old, remembers having "a hard time formulating thoughts and some of the things I said either didn't make sense or were jumbled in terms of syntax" (personal interview). Camila Parra Diaz, whose *migraña puzón* attacks began at age 13, recalls her brother's attacks, which began when he was six years old: "[M]y parents thought he'd been drugged. He was talking nonsense and didn't recognize anyone" (personal interview). Such prodromal features, combining speech, visual, and cognitive processing impairment, have led to some diagnosing this constellation of experiences as "confusional migraine."

Though pain is a private, even isolating, experience, David B. Morris writes that "politics is always subtly at work shaping how we experience pain" (146). The pain of child migraine is no different, though its politics are perhaps even less visible than the disorder itself. One common expectation, which causes neglect surrounding chronic pain syndromes, is that all pain will be observable. Helen Neal explains, "Complicating the pain control situation is the fact that physicians and nurses use manifestations of acute pain as the basis for judging all pain. Sudden, intense pain may produce observable changes in respiration, sweating, pulse rate, or pallor" but, a nurse tells her, "'When pain persists for hours or days, or sometimes even a few minutes, a process of adaptation occurs. Physiological parameters return to normal" (174–175). Pain is a much more complicated phenomenon than most would intuit (even to those suffering from chronic pain, like that from a phantom limb, their condition can seem counterintuitive—it simply makes no sense, often signifying only neural dysfunction). There are rampant misconceptions about pain that interfere with a painfree person's empathy. Most, if they have not learned otherwise, believe "[t]here is a correct amount of pain for a given injury" (Schechter 785). Some believe "that analgesia makes diagnosis difficult" with pediatric patients or "that opioid dose should relate to disease severity rather than pain intensity" (Cousins et al. 1). But no two people respond to the same pain stimulus in the same way or feel it to the same degree, and not all pain is nociceptive (a direct response to external, physically observable, or "real," stimuli, as in a visible wound, broken bone, or infected organ).

The problem of chronic pain is even more fraught with potential for misunderstanding, as it is invisible, especially in those most silenced of patients, such as children. In cases of dysfunctional pain (pain created in the brain or neuropathically instead of nociceptively—migraine includes both), self-report, especially from children, can be perceived with skepticism, disbelief, insistence that such pain is exaggerated, or even accusations of lying. In *The Culture of Pain*, David B. Morris writes, "It is not a pleasant trait, but we sometimes feel suspicious of people who say they are in pain but who do not groan or pound the floor. Pain patients know what it means to face daily suspicion" (68). Apparently this unsympathetic trait is not so much learned as it needs to be unlearned. In medical studies of child perceptions of pain, one of the most commonly identified causes attributed to it is punishment (see Ross 1984, Gafney and Dunne 1987, Hurley and Whelan 1988). Children often assume that others are in pain because they deserve it for some wrongdoing. The demand to legitimize through narrative for any understanding may begin on the playground.

Child migraineurs are invisibly disabled in that their pain is invisible, in fact, practically impossible to prove outwardly, and in the sense that they are marginalized and muted persons culturally. Making child migraine more visible requires breaking down common misconceptions about dysfunctional pain, child migraineurs, and impairments that remain so easily undetected. A contributing step in the right direction has come in the past three decades of research into pediatric pain, which have disproven the old myths that "[c]hildren's nervous systems are too immature to experience pain. . . . Children have no memory of pain. Children become easily addicted to narcotics" (Schechter 785). For some practitioners these were necessary illusions, created to make it psychologically easier to inflict pain on babies and children in order to save their lives when doctors lacked the necessary tools, research, or knowledge to manage their pain safely in any way but restraining them. The ideology that surrounded such myths, however, supported an institutional climate that was abusive toward the young. In 1980 Michael Rothenberg would write, "It is my conviction that children's hospitals are still run for the convenience of the adults who work in them, with only a secondary focus on the needs of the children treated in them" (22). Priscilla Alderson would write in 1993 of the British experience, that schools are even worse on this issue: "[C]hildren in hospital have certain autonomy rights, but schools deny basic rights to their pupils, and are imposing unprecedented amounts of compulsory tests and curriculum subjects on them. Parents, not children, are perceived as the consumers of education" (31). Two of the most powerful institutions shaping our children today still serve parents and adult workers before the children who are dependent upon them and whom they are meant to serve.

Melanie Thernstrom quotes one doctor as saying, "To value someone's suffering, you have to validate them as a person. We shouldn't be surprised that the least-valued members of society get the least pain relief" (166). Empathy for child pain has always coexisted with firm denials of it—though children may be valued sentimentally, their needs are not put first when those sentiments are threatened. Arthur Frank writes that "we see children only as what they will do when they become adults. . . . In children most of all we want to deny illness" (2002, 128). Our denial is enabled to perpetuate by the fact that a child in prolonged pain usually satisfies adult expectations for *good* child behavior—basically behaving in the opposite manner to a healthy child diagnosed with ADHD (attention-deficit hyperactivity disorder), for example—an experienced migraining child remains quiet, still, making no trouble. Consider the description of a young migraineur in Bille's (1962) study:

> From 2–4 years of age he . . . lay down on his bed of his own accord. It was considered that he was "very good." His parents suspected, however, that he had headaches, and at the age of 5 years he complained of them himself.
>
> (74)

Perhaps even worse, is that a child faced with frequent pain may be seen as actually incapable, an assumption expressed to the extreme in this doctor's comment from 1889: "The stupid looking lazy child who frequently suffers from headache at school . . . is well worthy of the solicitous attention of the school medical officer" (Hill 712). Worthy of attention, indeed, though for more compassionate reasons.

Inflexible customs and institutions fail to make room for us to figure out our own, individualized modes of functional thriving. The presumption of "normalcy" can be just as oppressive as impositions of "abnormality"—to break that false rubric requires not simply debunking but also fully decentering the privileged standard. N. Ann Davis has identified the "double-bind of invisible disability," explaining that

> [w]hen [impaired] individuals are not "seen" as disabled, it can be more difficult for them to secure the assistance or accommodation they need to function effectively. . . . Those whose disabilities[11] are invisible may also have to convince other people that they really are *disabled*, not seeking some special – unfair – advantage; thus, what they must do is meet a burden of proof.
>
> (154)

This burden means that invisible disability socially demands narratives—confessional explanations:

This can be an awkward and thoroughly unpleasant undertaking, especially in a society in which "tact" is often interpreted as compelling able-bodied persons to refrain from attending to, or commenting on, perceived disability, and one in which people shun and stigmatize persons they see as disabled as a defense against having to confront their own vulnerability.

(205)

In these cases, the invisibly "disabled" person's explanations are met with disbelief or stubborn attempts at amateur diagnoses that are disguised as help but really explain away the condition as a result of something the impaired person is doing wrong (Have you tried ginger? What about cutting your hair?). In the case of migraine, it is the lack of visible evidence rather than a visible mark of suffering that can enable condescension and neglect.

What Gaye Tuchman has said of ADHD is certainly true of migraine: "We do not live in an era when individuals are branded with a mark of neurological difference. . . . Invisibility means that both adults and children with AD/HD are unavoidably and unwittingly passing as neurologically normal" (4). Passing might sound easy, but it's not when you need help finding a quiet dark place to lie down and work or school completely disallows it. It's also not very helpful when you are trying to convince doctors how profoundly your quality of life is affected: "No one, except the person experiencing it, doubts the value of pain as a warning of something amiss, but its value depends on the availability of means for correcting it" (Neal 4). Melanie Thernstrom adds, "Part of the curse of pain is that it *sounds* untrue to people who don't have pain" (135). So, as Jean Jackson points out, "Pain is doubly paradoxical: It is a quintessentially private experience that depends on social action to make it real to others, yet that very same action can also arouse suspicions about its reality" (2005, 342). N. Ann Davis explains the logic (and motives) behind this paradox: "Because people with invisible disabilities appear to meet able-bodied standards, they are viewed as able-bodied: they 'pass.' Moreover, because they have passed, the revelation of their disability may seem, at some level, to be the revelation of prior deceit" (206). Because our impairments unpleasantly remind others that we all are likely to experience disability at some point in our lives,

> nondisabled persons are prone to both exaggerate the degree of difference between themselves and persons with disabilities and to suppose that . . . if someone is disabled, it will be obvious. People with invisible disabilities are thus often put in the position of having to rebut the presumption of "normalcy."
>
> (207)

So, protest and protest we must. Pathographies, medical ethnographies, and disability memoirs abound.

Like any identity politics surrounding difference, the politics of disability often require both greater recognition of categories and an equally passionate critique of that categorization. Susan Wendell writes that "recognition of impairment is crucial to the inclusion of people with chronic illnesses in disability politics," yet "[s]uspicion surrounds people with chronic illnesses" (23, 28). In the case of migraine there is a clear category of specifically shared experience, which is not simply an allopathically defined norm. Migraineurs have certainly existed as long as humanity itself (as known from our earliest writings), and the unique set of symptoms (aura, unilateral head pain, nausea/vomiting, photophobia/phonophobia) that sets us apart is distinct and irrefutable. Recent research suggests a common causal factor in sluggish digestion, concluding that "migraine appears not to be just an episodic event in an otherwise normal person," implying, of course, that it is a regular event in similarly *ab*normal persons. One of the dangers of overgeneralizing from diagnoses is the disappearance of individuals and the diversity of their experiences with that diagnosis. In *The Biopolitics of Disability*, David Mitchell and Sharon Snyder warn that

> diagnosis extrapolates the diagnostic object into symptom clusters wherein the particularities of conditions are lost on behalf of consolidating generalizable medical categories of public aberrancy. Here a patient's privacy is "protected" while the disparate nature of variable bodies constituting the classification is diluted or erased all together.
>
> (69)

Migraine can cause anything from mild vascular headaches treatable with ibuprofen to a bed-ridden existence in permanent pain. As with other spectrum disorders, impairment can range so widely that the diagnosis fails to specify individual experience. But there is a good reason many individuals may also find diagnosis a necessary tool toward understanding. Kristin Barker has written of how having an "illness narrative" and profile allows us to think of ourselves as belonging to a "unified illness identity" (279). By categorizing persons affected, we can forge common vocabularies and so recognize broader patterns of exclusion, including allopathically defined identity.

But many deny that this condition affects children as profoundly as it does adults (and I believe the social disability, the oppressive ramifications, for children to be much worse), because, as Andrew Levy points out, "most migraining children escape attention" (57). Some adults seem to take comfort in and overemphasize differential factors, such as the fact that child migraine attacks are generally shorter in duration than those of adults and sometimes present more as abdominal discomfort (cyclical vomiting) than excruciating head pain. Yet even in 1912 neurologist Martin Thiemich would point out that for children "the disease is in every respect so like the migraine of adults that we are justified in omitting a more detailed discussion" (quoted in Ashwal 603). So I have two seemingly contrary aims: to convincingly argue that indeed children suffer the same malady, but also to establish that the complications of being a child with this malady create a *unique* set of problems we must facilitate resolving. And I will argue that resistance isn't just found in rejecting medicalization—it is also found in negotiating awareness of disability politics into full advocacy *and* utilizing allopathic resources without being exploited.

I do not want to make the mistake of encouraging uncritical essentialization of child migraineurs, or migraineurs in general; however, in the fourth chapter I will rely heavily on testimonies from migraineurs of all ages about common bonds that can be found among us—after all, our shared physiological experiences shape certain responses and accommodation needs in common. And knowing we have a common bond can be immensely therapeutic. This is another paradox of invisible disability—we have to embrace *categorical* recognition[12] in order for our *individual* impairment to be taken seriously by a community that will accommodate customized needs and yet look beyond the very difference that has been used to define them. For this reason I opt to retain the term "migraineur"[13] rather than the "person first" language advised in social work and disability politics that would sanction using "person with migraine." I noticed in my interviews with fellow "persons with migraine" that when I carelessly dropped the term "migraineur," many seemed to pick it up in a sense that indicated political solidarity.

There is a positive outcome to all of the compulsive confessionals demanded of invisibly impaired individuals—circulating stories is an effective way of creating a sense of community. Such narratives help us to connect, or at least feel connected, to others who experience the same impairments and might make sense of them, imparting positive coping strategies. This function is one of many reasons for the importance of Myra Bluebond-Langner's milestone ethnography, *The Private Worlds of Dying Children* (1978), in which she manages, through the more "objective" scientific methods of anthropology to collect the voices of children with leukemia, while actually *telling their stories* with attention to their subjective experiences. By adopting a dramatic format she turns her observations into "a composite play," through which we can experience what she learned within a personalized context rather than simply following an accumulation of isolated perspectives. Whereas Bluebond-Langner developed a literary rhetoric from anthropological data, I incorporate an interdisciplinarily inspired, informal ethnographic set of "data" into my rhetorical and literary analysis. To do so I interviewed 30 current and former child-migraineurs (and some parents) over a period of six years, whose stories are integrated to help provide concrete impressions of living with migraine; but I also, in keeping with my background in language and literature, incorporate accounts from literary and popular sources to indicate the layered pervasiveness of disabling patterns in social discourse.

I hope to provide a larger but simultaneously concrete picture of how child migraineurs live, hurt, cope, and negotiate the burdens of invisible disability, which in turn can effect a sense of solidarity that is healing. Arthur Frank writes, "The ill body's articulation in stories is a personal task, but the stories told by the ill are also *social*" (1995, 3). This book, I hope, is a social act. In my next two chapters I will historically contextualize the disabling social forces and discursive patterns that continue to exacerbate the individual impaired experience of child migraineurs, then in following chapters I will attempt to re-create the sense of community I gained in doing my research—through recognizing actual voices of migraineurs and by investigating the myriad ways in which society has tried to ignore or tame their pain.

Notes

1 Mervyn J. Eadie indicates that "ancient and medieval authors nearly always dealt with headache in general, or with types of headache that do not correspond at all closely with the modern categories of the disorder," but the "classic" combination of symptoms has been consistently reported and represented in every age (113).

2 This is not to say that migraine is the same as other disabilities or even that the oppression is simply analogous, but that the impairment is considered far more seriously by health professionals than the general public would guess. Through the blending of social and phenomenological models exemplified by Jill C. Humphrey, Susan Wendell, and Margaret Price, disability studies has come to include, even break down, former distinctions of healthy/unhealthy, acute/chronic, even disabled/nondisabled and mental/physical, which makes it an immensely informative discourse from which to consider migraine.

3 See Bille (1962, 44, 48), Sillanpää (1983, 15), Abu-Arefeh (1994, 767), and Antilla et al. (2006, e1199).

4 Likewise, in the case of ADHD, "[e]ndless studies that find children are hyperactive at home but not at school, or at summer camp (where 40 percent of the population was on chronic prescription drugs in 2006) but not in clinicians' rooms, do serious disservice to biological claims" (T. Miller 146). However, in the case of migraine, though school is the predominant stressor (not cause), children also get the attacks from pleasant stressors, like birthday parties, sports, and summer camp.

5 Migraine, as diagnosed by Vahlquist and Bille, is an episodic paroxysmal headache "accompanied by at least two of the following features: unilaterality, nausea, visual aura, and family history of migraine" (Lipton, 231). It is since understood that "[u]nilaterality is less common in pediatric migraine than in adult migraine," abdominal symptoms can predominate head pain in children, aura is actually experienced by a minority of migraineurs, and also that nonheredity cannot be seen as an excluding factor (232). According to current International Headache Society standards, or ICHD-II, the diagnosed subject must have two of the following: pulsating, unilateral, moderate to severe pain that is lessened with inactivity – accompanied by nausea or photophobia and phonophobia.

6 Though the schools remained similar environments within these consistent samples, "in the districts of the city with the highest social instability" both prevalence and incidence were greater (Sillanpää and Antilla 1996, 466). Again the importance of environmental variables is indicated: "From the age of 4 years, the curve was markedly higher and steeper in 1992 than in 1974," increasing "from 1.9% to 5.7% (468).

7 Processed foods, hidden food allergy, and even fatty foods have been implicated as migraine triggers (Bic 1999, Alpay 2010). Early stages of research (funded, however, by GlaxoSmithKline) into fat cell biomarkers suggest that "a protein hormone secreted from fat tissue and known to modulate several of the pain pathways is implicated in migraine. The hormone is also implicated in sugar metabolism, insulin regulation, immunity and inflammation, as well as obesity, which is a risk factor for migraines" (Desmon 2013).

8 Here's the self-help genre in a nutshell: commonly used supplements include feverfew (recommended as an ancient remedy), vitamin B-2 (riboflavin), magnesium, butterbur, 5-HTP, and L-Tryptophan. Knowing how to activate acupuncture point P6 with pressure may help with nausea: "two finger-breadths below the wrist, right between the two prominent tendons of the lower arm" (Enders 104–105). Ginger also helps (juiced, drops in juice, sublingual, or capsules). If not, opt for suppository antinausea meds rather than oral when possible – they are kid friendly, will be more effective, and do less damage to the liver.

9 Ha-Joon Chang writes of the "knowledge economy" myth pursued in the United States, assuming that high academic performance increases or is even correlated with a nation's

productivity and wealth, arguing instead that standardized, heavily assessed education is merely about "sorting" (186). Students get unnecessary college degrees in countries that ascribe to the myth: "The higher education system in these countries has become like a theatre in which some people decided to stand to get a better view, prompting others behind them to stand. Once enough people stand, everyone has to stand, which means that no one is getting a better view, while everyone has become more uncomfortable" (188).

10 In addition to multiple chemical sensitivities, Chen also experienced migraine as a youth: "The migraines announced themselves with a visual signature: if I looked just to the left of someone, I could make that person simply disappear, amid shifting zipper lines within my field of vision. Soon after this aura came the extraordinary pain, and then came the sequence of rolling migraines. My visits to doctors and acupuncturists, my ingestion of meds, and my otherwise widespread attempts did little to stem the tide of migraines" (2014, 172).

11 Among the impairments Davis includes as potentially invisible disabilities are rheumatoid arthritis, multiple prostheses, CFS (198), severe depression, chronic pain, PTSD, violent allergies, seizure disorders, severe fibromyalgia, MTBI, Crohn's disease, severe hypertension, degenerative joint disease, panic disorders, and chronic migraine (202). Davis qualifies: "There are many individuals with conditions, illnesses, and structural or biochemical anomalies that are life limiting but not readily discernible to others. . . . [who] may all appear 'normal' to people with whom they have casual interactions. Yet they may still be disabled: the quality of their lives may be no less profoundly or adversely impacted by these conditions" (153–154). Susan Wendell includes the following as what she calls "unhealthy" disabilities (as opposed to stabilized and healthy impaired conditions): "rheumatoid arthritis, fibromyalgia, lupus, ME/CFIDS, migraine headache, MS, and depression" (24).

12 This often misunderstood process, of typing in order to gain social change, is consistent with what Gayatri Chakravorty Spivak has called "strategic essentializing." Paddy Ladd effectively argues that deaf culture demonstrates the necessity of group identity in enabling individual freedoms within disability politics (275–276).

13 For an excellent analysis of the political precariousness of these terms, see Joanna Kempner (102–103). In his discussion of autism, Stuart Murray further nuances the implications of such language by contrasting "having autism" with "being autistic" that has fascinating implications about the way we identify our relationships to impairments through our identifiers. "Having" an impairment can suggest, positively, "that there is an independence from the disability" or, negatively, a rejection of solidarity with others similarly impaired (24). It could be seen as reifying a disease model uncritically embracing "cures," as well as encouraging denial of our shared animal vulnerabilities – refusing the knowledge that all of us will face impairment in our lives and can act more humanely, more proactively healthful being aware of that vulnerability and connectedness to others. "Being" impaired "conflates the person and the condition, and assumes that there is no possibility to move out of such a conflation" (24). Ultimately, Murray concludes, "I would like to think it is acceptable to be autistic, that it in fact illuminates a way of being human" (24). Likewise I believe one can *be* a migraineur without being a stigma, a stereotype, or reduced to representing migraine itself.

2 A history of pediatric pain and the politics of pill culture

"As a kid, you don't know why you are in intense pain. It's the most terrifying experience a child can have. There's no reason for it, and some may feel it is punishment. I don't think I'll ever get over the fear of that kind of pain."

Caleb Hood

Tobin Siebers wrote in 2008 that "the greatest stake in disability studies at the present moment is to find ways to represent pain and to resist models of the body that blunt the political effectiveness of these representations" (61). Nowhere is this burden more uniformly clear than in our treatment of young people living with disability or disease. Our insistence that they remain manageable and undemanding has resulted in a deep ideological refusal to recognize pediatric pain as an imperative call for relief. Though pain relief has become globally recognized as a basic human right (Janeti and Liebeskind 1994, Cousins et al. 2004, Brennan et al. 2007, Gwyther et al. 2009, Macpherson 2009, Dahler 2010)—and, incidentally, Michael J. Cousins even includes treatment of dysfunctional pain like migraine explicitly in the consideration of as such a fundamental right (2000)—this right is not consistently extended to include children in practice.

Many have rallied to recognize children's basic rights to pain relief (Walco et al. 1994, Mack and Wolfe 2006, Marston 2011). But historically child pain has only gone from untreated to undertreated, and "when the court is asked to decide, decisions about the appropriate treatment of young children . . . are made with regard to the future but without consideration of the present reality of life for the child" (Bridgeman 2002). The present reality of a child's life can be debilitating pain— a reality that adult-centered prejudice allows us to deny in the cruelest of ways (Marston 2011). Recent evidence of this prejudice surrounds responses to the Food and Drug Administration's approval of OxyContin for use in children in October of 2015. Hillary Rodham Clinton, who has past legal expertise in child welfare and should know better, responded that the decision was "absolutely incomprehensible" (Saint Louis). One might suspect that her disapproval stemmed from the need to regulate the pharmaceutical industry and curb the profit motive that leads to fraudulently prescribing drugs off-label[1] in order to redress the therapeutic orphaning of ill children through undertesting. After all, the irony is that the same protectionism that keeps children from being test subjects in most drug studies also hinders the development of drugs that might protect them from disease or relieve pain more safely. But Clinton's response was classic, knee-jerk opiophobia and protectonism. Dr. Kathleen A. Neville, a pediatric oncologist, rebutted simply, "Come be one of my kids whose pelvis gets eaten out by cancer," voicing the reality our discourse tends to silence (Saint Louis). Kids can suffer, immensely, and just refusing to acknowledge that suffering does nothing to relieve it.

Rather than productively regulating uncommissioned research on drugs in development and reducing the power corporations hold to escalate costs that make drugs inaccessible to all but the rich, popular discourse surrounding pharmaceuticals and children tends to dredge up the worst of our reductive assumptions: kids are junkies just waiting for that first taste, or they don't need the hard stuff anyway. And if we look a little deeper at our cultural biases, there is always underlying fear for children's welfare getting in the way of actually ensuring it. *New York Times* reporter Judith Warner writes, in her book *We've Got Issues*, that "the Medicated Child is the trope that brings together all of our diffuse worries about childhood in our day" (173). Indeed, at the beginning of the twenty-first century, panic culture surrounded the medicated child, largely in relation to ADHD medications and more recently over vaccinations—but less sensationalized, and seemingly irreconcilable, concerns have surrounded children, popular discourse, medical practice, and school policy for the last three decades in a completely contradictory manner that reveals much older ideological roots. In this chapter I expose the historical silencing of child pain in the public imagination that has enabled continuing neglect of child pain. Tracing the current state of twisted logic that results in overmedicating children for undesirable behaviors yet undertreating their pain back through previous centuries, I will suggest a concurrent development in education, wherein zero-tolerance, assessment-focused bureaucracy has resulted in a powerful edu-pharmaceutical complex, selectively medicating children where it befits adult control.

Take the 1984 Reagan campaign as an exemplary entry point to historically contextualizing these agendas. As Rosalind P. Petchesky recounts, "Beginning with the 1984 presidential campaign, the neoconservative Reagan administration and the Christian Right accelerated their use of television and video imagery to capture political discourse—and power" (264). This media campaign would include the use of the 1984 antiabortion film *The Silent Scream*, which used the silent scream trope to encapsulate fetal pain and effect an emotional response in viewers. Mary S. Sheridan explains, "Many of those opposed to abortion buttress their argument with description of the excruciating death of the fetus" (88). This rhetorical method wasn't a protest against fetal pain but an attempt to punish would-be but unwilling mothers. Its reasoning would later inspire the proposed 2005 Unborn Child Pain Awareness Act, which, Alissa Perrucci explains, would have "required physicians performing abortions at or after twenty weeks of gestation to read a script . . . wherein the physician must offer the patient pain medication for the fetus. . . . Situated within the language of this script, a patient refusing fetal pain medication would appear to be something akin to a sociopath," even though the extra anesthetic endangered the pregnant woman (138–139). From approximately 1978 through the 1980s, the silent scream trope dominated prolife propaganda, but not once did it result in awareness of how little attention was paid to fetal, neonatal, infant, toddler, or child pain in general. Instead, as Keith Wailoo writes, pain ultimately "became a symbol for Reagan of the dependence, the learned helplessness, and the growth of government that conservatives so detested" (128). In fact, those wrapped in the rhetoric seem to have been entirely ignorant of the medical norms for treating actual young, unborn and born, bodies in pain.

Though rhetorically the silent scream trope might have seemed to help advocate for greater sensitivity to the pain of the young, the agenda behind it reveals actual indifference. Former congressman Barney Frank famously quipped that "profamily" neoconservatives act "as if life begins at conception and ends at birth" (Pogrebin 47). The disconnection between political lip service and any actual defense of the young is too easily overlooked. For example, Michael Rothenberg wrote in the same time period that the results in Washington were representative: "Within 18 months after passing a mandatory child abuse reporting law, the State Legislature, as part of an overall economy drive cut the budget for Children's Protective Services in the State by 50 percent" (15). Another physician would likewise point to such a disconnection in our commitment to child welfare: "We spend more health care dollars per person in the last week of life than in the previous seventy-five years . . . and with much less pay off" (quoted in Pogrebin 50). Many Americans remain oblivious to our dismal performance in the global context, but generally put, "The health of U.S. children is worse in virtually all categories when compared to children in other industrialized countries" (Starfield 2004).

During the time in which the silent scream trope galvanized and was bandied about by the religious right, less sensationalized changes were occurring in terms of publically recognizing neonate pain, changes which ultimately were far more profound in their impact on actual treatment. In 1985 the unanaesthetized surgeries of premature neonate Jeffrey Lawson (to be discussed in more detail later) would prompt mother Jill Lawson to expose what the religious right was clearly oblivious to in their indignant propaganda against what they claimed to see as medical indifference to fetal pain: that even neonate pain was medically unrecognized and untreated at the time. Pediatrician Lonnie K. Zeltzer explains,

> I can hardly believe that until the late 1980s it was commonly accepted in the medical world that children do not feel pain in the same way that adults do. In fact, during my training, it was common practice to rationalize that infants do not feel pain, but that even if they do, they don't remember it. So it was that infants underwent major surgery without anesthesia and no postoperative pain medication. Often they would be given a medication that would paralyze them but leave them fully aware of the pain. I remember learning to perform circumcisions on newborns during my pediatric training while they were strapped to what was called a papoose board. I watched, horrified, as their little faces turned beet red and they screamed their heads off.

(1)

Speechless?

If you are thinking that such withholding of drugs from newborns reflects the general antidrug climate of the time, think again. A similar disconnection between political discourse, public opinion, and medical practices occurred with the Reagan administration's use of drug-war rhetoric. In 1985, Nancy Reagan's "Just Say No" campaign was peaking and going international, advocating a simplistic position that kids could "just say no" to drugs, that is, controlled substances. Meanwhile schools and collaborating doctors were prescribing performance-enhancing drugs, that is, controlled substances, to children at rates never seen before. In the case of Ritalin alone, "[i]n 1970, 150,000 children were using it, increasing to 900,000 in 1990" (147). In the 1990s the use of Ritalin would increase by 1,700% (Diller, 52). Eventually, off-label, these numbers would grow to include toddlers—most recent estimates have "10,000 American toddlers" medicated for ADHD (Schwartz). In the midst of such changes, Jane Gross would ask, "How has it come to pass that in fin-de-siècle America, where every child from preschool onward can recite the 'anti-drug' catechism by heart, millions of middle- and upper-middle class children are being legally drugged with a substance so similar to cocaine that, as one journalist accurately summarized the science, 'it takes a chemist to tell the difference'?" (*New York Times* July 16, 2006). I hope to plumb some answers to this question in contextualizing child migraine.

The mid to late 1980s was only the beginning of what would be seen as a child epidemic (along with obesity) at the turn of the century, but the fact that it was only the beginning speaks to how disconnected such discourses are. Judith Warner writes that "what the often outsized vitriol makes clear is that the passion is ideological and only tangentially about real children" (4). Conflicting agendas have been clashing, with real children left behind in the nonsensical fallout. How is it that in theory and sentiment we can so right-mindedly recognize injustices against the young, but in policy and practice go so wrong? In the interrelated strains of discourse just mentioned, the only connecting logic is the common desire to control women and children, a willingness to exploit their medical vulnerabilities, and using them for sentimental appeals that belie an actual lack of concern for the persons in question. In each case a party identifies an injustice against the young bodies of those who cannot advocate on their own behalf, proceeds to speak for them, and in doing so, often, perhaps with good intentions, tramples their rights and "best interests."

Even antiabortion activists who invoke the "right to life" ultimately avoid using the rhetoric or reasoning of human rights discourse in their arguments. Of more politically objective treatments, on the issue of fetal pain (Tessa Richards) or fetal rights (Alston, Cornock, and Montgomery), those arguing are limited by the legal limitations of applying human rights for the fetus by legal definitions of "a person." The reality is that until birth, advocacy for the fetus depends entirely upon adult projection. Anyone arguing about fetal medical rights comes up against the same obstacle to authority that pro-lifers invoked as proof of their own by protesting too much. As John T. Noonan Jr. would write,

[O]ur normal way of knowing whether someone is in pain is for the person to use language affirming that he or she is suffering. . . . Infants, the unborn, and animals[2] have no conceptual language in which to express their suffering and its degree.

(205)

In fact, learning to "read" infant pain involves learning how to recognize nonverbal cues, the most powerful of which is frequently downplayed but, Mary S. Sheridan points out, usually presents at birth: "It is ironically true that pain validates an infant's humanity: a baby's first cry is the sign of its life as an independent being" (86). I'd tweak this insight slightly—the cry confirms that the baby is alive, but the scream of pain remains connected with basic animal expression, gradually stifled through socialization to be accepted into the human community. Perhaps adults silence screams and cries, not just out of sympathy and instinctive concern, but to deny the animal vulnerability of our own bodies.

The infant's cry is an effective pain response when the stimulus is acute and straightforward, but the history of medical practice has long-established ways of avoiding the confrontation of that cry, and not all pain is acute or nociceptive (responding to a traceable stimulus), which further facilitates denial. There is also a strong silencing effect in habituation and socialization, as David B. Morris explains, in *The Culture of Pain*:

> All newborn infants cry, and their cries (as all parents know) come in distinctively different tones. Yet this apparently natural response to pain – although not itself learned – is swiftly unlearned and relearned. We very soon replace our earliest natural responses to pain with carefully calibrated understandings about how much crying is permitted, about when and where you can cry, about who can cry and for what reasons. . . . We learn almost everything we know about pain, including the need to deny it and to smother it in silence.
>
> (72)

The newborn's cry is only briefly heard and celebrated as a sign of life in films, for example, but anything beyond it is suppressed—uncontrolled screaming, ironically, is rendered unspeakable to squelch our own sense of helplessness at understanding what it communicates. In literature, which is almost entirely complicit in the rhetorical silencing of child pain, an exception to the rule is seen in the death of Monsieur Othon's son in *The Plague* (1947), by Albert Camus. His departure from the norm is to focus entirely upon the wails of a boy dying from the plague. And the noise incites protest:

> [S]lowly the lips parted and from them rose a long, incessant scream, hardly varying with his respiration, and filling the ward with a fierce, indignant protest, so little childish that it seemed like a collective voice issuing from all the sufferers there. . . . But the wail continued without cease and the other sufferers began to grow restless. The patient at the far end of the ward, whose little broken cries had gone on without a break, now quickened their tempo so that they flowed together in one unbroken cry.
>
> (194–195)

Notably, when Camus represents migraine, in his later story, "The Growing Stone," from *Exile and the Kingdom* (1957), his adult male protagonist's pain is elevated to the level of a Sisyphean struggle, though stoically endured.

In telling contrast to the consciously corporeal experiences represented in Camus is the dominant Western sentimental tradition of silent suffering that characterizes one of the most prominent uses of child figures in earlier American fiction, especially, most famously exemplified by the gentle, quiet, and angelic deaths of Little Eva in *Uncle Tom's Cabin* (1852) or Beth in *Little Women* (1868). These fictional devices are not simply reflections of nineteenth-century sentimentality but an ideological legacy that has resulted in deeply rooted biases of our own time—norms that are oppressively based on adult denial of children's pain and their right to relief. Even when child characters are given something to dampen their pain, like the eponymous heroine in *Pollyanna* (1913), who is swiftly given "little white pills" when she awakens from an accident paralyzed and hurting (168–169), there are hints that it is done more for the sake of adults around them than for the child. Pollyanna's nurse knows "that her patient must be *quieted . . .* and she now stood at the bedside with the *quieting powder* ready" (my ital, 186). What we often overlook in such public sentiments surrounding childhood are the adult motives of denial, silencing pain or its expression, and the more disturbing instruments of using it to keep children in control.

The silenced scream

Long before the trope of the silent scream emerged, over a century and a half of complicated relations between doctors and patients in pain would lead to the ultimate silencing of child pain as a normal part of treatment in the twentieth-century United States. Knowing how and why we got to that point is one goal of my analysis, but to understand why these questions are important to children's medical, literary, and disability history, I first want to show how recent and pervasive the denial of neonate pain has been in order to get a realistic comprehension of the longer-standing legacy of child pain. The most famous exemplification of the cause came in the case of Jeffrey Lawson.

On February 9, 1985, Jeffrey Lawson was born at 25–26 weeks of age (five weeks older than the fetal subjects of the 1980s antiabortion rhetoric). Born so prematurely, he needed much medical intervention through procedures for which his mother was assured he would be anesthetized. After Jeffrey's death at two weeks, Jill Lawson found through his medical records that

> Jeffrey had holes cut on both sides of his neck, another hole cut in his chest, an incision from his breastbone around to his backbone, his ribs pried apart, and an extra artery near his heart tied off with another hole cut in his left side for a chest tube. The operation lasted one and a half hours. Jeffrey was awake through it all. The anesthesiologist paralyzed him with Pavulon, a curare drug that left him unable to move, *but totally conscious.*
>
> (Jill Lawson, emp in original, 125)

There will be many anecdotes throughout this book meant to illustrate extremes. The case of Jeffrey Lawson is not one of them. For you to understand how standard the acceptance of neonate pain was as an inevitable yet untreatable byproduct of surgical procedures (life- and non-life-saving), you need to understand that Jeffery Lawson's case represented the norm. Helen Harrison, in 1986, listed unanesthetized infant procedures such as "major surgery, chest tube insertions, cutdowns (all performed without painkillers); gangrene and amputations from infiltrated IVs; bones broken during chest physiotherapy: skin pulled off with adhesive tape; burns from the monitors" (124). She reports parental responses, like that of one mother: "[I]f this were going on in any other setting . . . it would be called torture" (124). Another "noted the similarity between the aversive behavior of some NICU babies and the psychologic problems of adult torture victims" (124). Harrison recounts another parent who "realized anesthesia would not be used for her daughter's surgery [and] refused to sign the consent form. The operation was performed anyway and the mother was reported to local authorities[3] as an abusive parent" (124). Harrison concludes, "In the past two decades a great deal has been written about parents as abusers of their premature babies. The time has now come for a long, hard look at the *medical* abuse of newborns" (124). During the next decade, activism, scholarship, and medical research led to reforms in treating pediatric pain, especially operative pain, particularly in neonates, yet Jeffrey Lawson's case helps to demonstrate the inertia of medical tradition and the willing naïveté of an uninitiated general public.

How, in the 1980s, were such practices still the norm? The answers to this question help also to contextualize the cultural silencing of children's invisible pains as well. As Patrick J. McGrath and Anita M. Unruh have put it, "Public pressure is a very crude method to trigger change. Public pressure does not distinguish between well-validated scientific finding and quack medicine or speculation" (564). The sentimental appeals and imperfect public understanding of medical practices will be the subject of my investigation—mining deep historical biases that don't add up in order to expose embedded premises that have enabled injustices to become norms. Public discourse reveals much about how and why we justify or disregard child pain.

Influential scholars in the humanities (Elaine Scarry, Martin S. Pernick, David B. Morris) tried to grasp pain theoretically in the mid-1980s to early 1990s, and in their work we can find some explanations of why only recently rights to pain control have been, selectively, extended to children. Power over pain itself has been historically suspect and slowly accepted. Suffering was alternately seen as religiously purifying or divine punishment, in either case, not to be altered by scientific intervention. Martin S. Pernick also records a bias in some physicians for the nineteenth-century concept of "counterirritation," by which one is cured from one disease by another, or one pain cancels another:

> The theory that pain is therapeutic reflected overtones of older beliefs – medicine must be painful to be effective because nothing of value can be attained

without suffering. Pain constitutes one of the oldest measures of value, a connection still expressed by the dual connotations of words like *labor* and *painstaking*. The word *indolent* now means "lazy," but in medical terminology it retains its original meaning, "painless."

(45)

Frank Brennen et al. recount that "[t]he word *patient* itself is derived from the Latin *patiens*, meaning 'one who suffers'" (208). These beliefs might seem very outdated by today's standards, but they remain influential in the victim-blaming of the invisibly impaired. And in the United States, palliative care has been widely deprioritized far below diagnostic troubleshooting: "The determinative principle of responsible medical care is not 'Do no *hurt*.' It is 'Do no *harm*'" (Walco et al. 2003, 159). In the United States, such beliefs persisted and circulated long after their consolatory necessity.

In European history, not all religious inflections on pain were punishing, as Esther Cohen contextualizes: "The main business of twelfth-century saints was health. From the thirteenth century onward, the function of alleviation was added to healing" (205). In fact, Cohen writes of French practices that

[b]y the fifteenth century, physicians were paying far more attention to pain . . . French physicians began using the word *mal* with its negative connotations, rather than the more neutral *doulour*, while the use of *peine* with its punitive connotations disappears from medical texts altogether.

(208)

As historians make clear, global debates about child pain, and especially infant pain, have always ranged between currently familiar extremes, yet the applications of anesthetics varied much in practice before the twentieth century. On one hand were romantic appeals in humanitarian responses, affected sentimentally, like that of seventeenth-century Swiss physician Felix Wurtz, who asked,

If a new skin in old people be tender, what is it you think in a new born Babe? Doth a small thing pain you so much on a finger, how painful is it then to a Child, which is tormented all the body over, which hath but tendergrown flesh? If such a perfect Child is tormented so soon, what shall we think of a Child, which stayed not in the wombe its full time? Surely it is twice worse with him.

(Ruhrah 204–205)

The ethical concerns about authority to act on the infant's behalf were certainly recognized as medical expertise developed, as indicated by Andrew O'Malley, who writes of the British context,

One of the common objections to professionalizing pediatric medicine in the eighteenth century was that infants were incapable of informing physicians of what ailed them. Acquiring the necessary information to formulate a diagnosis relied on the verbal communication of the patient, and since infants could not perform this function, perhaps leaving their medical care to the mothers and nurses most familiar with them was the best course.

(81)

But the results were not always in the best interests of individualized children:

> [F]ar from being the least treatable of patients, the mute infant becomes the ideal medical subject, one in whom the signs and symptoms are given their fiercest expression, unhampered by potentially inaccurate or contradictory spoken communication. . . . The children become the disease from which they suffer, reduced to a description of the symptoms they display.

(82)

The inability of young patients to advocate for their own medical interests has historically complicated progress in developing consistent, effective, or humane treatment.

In the United States, both punishing and silencing rhetoric persisted in the treatment of the young. During the nineteenth century, which Martin S. Pernick calls the "Age of Pain," radical changes occurred—the primary opiates were isolated for consistently dosable use, the hypodermic syringe was invented and rapidly utilized widely, and anesthesia by inhalation was introduced—empowering surgeons and physicians: "this direction to decide who shall suffer and who shall be relieved constituted an enormous source of power for the physician, in maintaining authority and control over the patient" (139). Initially there was resistance to anesthetizing the youngest patients:

> The degree of sensitivity in children proved an especially controversial issue. Dr. Abel Pierson of Massachusetts declared that infants could sleep insensibly even while undergoing surgery. Pierson, Henry J. Bigelow, and others who believed in infant insensibility, assumed that the ability to experience pain was related to intelligence, memory, and rationality; like the lower animals, the very young lacked the mental capacity to suffer.

(150)

But, "As the idea that 'women[4] and children' comprised a single category gained popularity in Romantic Era America, the view that young children were extremely vulnerable to pain came to dominate" (150). However, early use of anesthetics on infants and children seems to have been motivated much less by sympathy or recognition of nonconsent and vulnerability than a practical convenience—anesthetized patients are easier to control. Whereas with older patients, their consciousness might allow them to assist surgeons with ongoing reports as to their status, infants were incapable of report, and so their consciousness was unnecessary. Thus, as Pernick reports,

For children too little to be restrained by reason, yet too big to be restrained easily by force, anesthesia was especially valuable. . . . [T]he combination of high sensitivity to pain, difficulty in managing the patient, and ease of anesthetization made children from about two years old to adolescence unexcelled subjects for the use of anesthetics.

(172–173)

Note that infants here were already factored out of considerations for anesthesia due to the ease of restraint in spite of higher sensitivity to pain, a practice that would continue into the late 1970s and early 1980s in the use of "papoose" boards customized for the purpose.

By the mid-nineteenth century, anesthesia would become more widespread for child patients undergoing operations; in fact, Pernick reports that by this time they received more anesthesia than older patients: "[C]hildren got anesthesia much more frequently than did adults undergoing non-capital surgery. Children under ten got anesthetics in four out of every five such operations; only half of the adolescents and young adults received ether" (191). Again, the consistent motivating factor was manageability, control. Pernick, whose valuable mining of historical medical sources produced plentiful evidence, provides these pertinent examples. First, "[t]he Massachusetts General Hospital's Dr. Samuel Cabot, Jr. revealed what he saw to be the central purpose in anesthetizing infants when he noted of one 1854 operation that the young patient had been 'rolled firmly in a sheet as a substitute for ether'" (229). In another case from 1857,

the frustrated physician decided against the use of anesthetics on a disruptive young child[5] with a dislocated thigh: "I determined to let him suffer a while, in order to impress upon his mind more forcibly the necessity of keeping quiet."

(139)

As the sentimental valuation of children increased during the twentieth century (Viviana Zelizer), understandable concerns prevented doctors from taking the same risks they would with older patients. In addition, David Courtwright et al. explain that "[f]rom the early 1920s until the middle 1960s American narcotic policy was unprecedentedly strict and punitive" (1). Anesthetizing the youngest patients was seen as riskiest—logically among doctors because of fears of uncontrolled respiratory depression, illogically among the public because of fears of addiction. So, in the period that Barbara Ehrenreich and Deidre English would call "The Century of the Child," "with the public recognition of the special needs of children, the door was potentially opened to public responsibility for meeting those needs. . . . very little of this promise was realized" (166). Infants required greater doses of narcotic to be effective, but the conservative approach, especially to operating on infants, was a move toward paralyzing the patient without anesthesia or very little: "Altered drug metabolism and excretion resulting from immature excretory pathway often render neonates more susceptible to the respiratory depressant effects of opioids" (Bhatt-Mehta 1996, 764). Schechter et al.

(1986, 14) and Kuttner (2010, 27) claim these risks, however, have usually been exaggerated and can be countered with careful monitoring. Nevertheless, once paralyzing agents were developed and tested enough (even though there were many misgivings voiced about curare among doctors in print), pain control was dropped in practice, again showing that the nineteenth-century tactic of restraint was still the primary goal, not relieving infant pain. Paralyzing young subjects rather than treating pain was standard procedure for most of the twentieth century.

Jeffrey Lawson's neonatologist described surgery with only muscle relaxants and minimal anesthesia as "ignorance, hubris, and barbarism" (McGrath and Unruh 2002, 561). How could "barbarism" become standard procedure? For one thing, protectionism created an ethical dilemma in which children are protected from the medical testing that would develop treatments for them, thus leaving children untreatable or treated without adequate testing for safety (dubbing them "therapeutic orphans" in the 1970s, which is highly relevant to the dilemma of child migraineurs today). But we have a much longer history of taking advantage of the pain of vulnerable others: "Parents use pain to discipline. Theologians preach its spiritual values" (Neal 94). The threat of pain is ubiquitously used even in our anti–corporal punishment climate. To some it may seem unavoidable. Gary Walco et al. report that the nineteenth-century view of counterirritation is still sometimes grasped as an excuse: "[U]nrelieved pain is necessary to gain something better" (2003, 157). Pain in young persons can be easier to overlook than we acknowledge—and doctors likewise can avoid noticing: "It is a contradiction that most of us do not notice—we routinely impose pain on sick and vulnerable infants" (McGrath and Unruh 556). Some of this deniability comes from socialization; some from intuition that requires a rational override in cases where pain is difficult to read:

> Healthy neonates enjoy eye contact, vocalizing, and physical cuddling with their parents and their nurses. The responsiveness of the neonate encourages increased social attention and nurturance on the part of parents and healthcare professionals and increases the probability of attending to the neonate's communication about pain. An ill neonate may have very little capability to engage in social exchanges.
>
> (McGrath and Unruh 558)

Especially when the pain is persistent, it is actually likely to create a listless patient less able to get required attention through interpersonal cues. As a result, Anand and Craig write, "the fact that the neonate's expression of unpleasantness does not fit within the strict definition of pain (imposed by the requirement for self-report) contributes to the failure to recognize and aggressively treat pain in infancy and early childhood" (5). This difficulty of reading pain applies as the baby grows: "[I]f an infant experiences severe pain exacerbated by any movement, then after first crying, the infant may become very still, neither moving or kicking, and may even stop crying to protect the painful area and conserve energy" (Kuttner 116). Many pain conditions, like migraine (which has been diagnosed in patients as young as four months), prevent the pain responses we intuitively respond to (anyone with chronic pain knows this double bind all too well). And in such cases, short of the power of articulation and verbal persuasion, a child is extremely disadvantaged.

The guilt and even empathy of adults for children in pain can also reinforce downplaying symptoms. Young children who present medical difficulties will internalize the frustration, guilt, and sometimes indifference around them. Chronic illness, in particular, can be such a constant influence that young patients will interpret themselves as burdens and feel the pressure to conform to adult ideals of painfree, healthy childhood. Cindy Dell Clark was told, by a chronically ill five-year old during doll play, "[E]verybody hates me when I'm sick" (153). This child was clearly demonstrating an early awareness of the social pressures to be "healthy" and the social stakes of being ill. Arthur W. Frank explains,

> An ill child withdraws when he senses that people do not like what he represents. To his parents he embodies their failure to have a healthy child. . . . To other children his presence brings a fear of something they understand only enough to worry that it will happen to them.
>
> (2002, 125)

Even when a child is receiving excellent medical and parental care, the anxieties of caretakers, guilt of frustrated doctors, and fears of other children can reinforce the notion that one is cast aside, and withdrawing is seldom interpreted as an expression of pain.

We also may easily overlook the social reinforcement of stoic attitudes in children from an early age. Helen Neal writes,

> If a child has not been raised in the stoical tradition, he quickly learns that it is expected of him in the hospital. Even a child suffering severely, when too tired to cry or rock or complain, will drop into an exhausted sleep, misleading those about him into thinking that his pain could not have been too bad.
>
> (174–175)

Coping skills develop early from necessity, but often they are hardly enough, and combined with an adult predisposition to downplay child pain, they can interfere with getting appropriate pain control. Mary S. Sheridan writes that some mistakenly believe that

> [c]hildren recover more quickly from painful procedures than adults do. It is true that children become more active more quickly than adults, but this may be because they use play, rather than words, as a distraction and thus a coping mechanism.
>
> (90)

Child resilience is a great asset, but unexpressed pain must also somehow be detected accurately and treated.

Some denial of child pain (or pain in general) has been historically necessary to practice medicine and maintain concentration. Martin Pernick describes how the ability to inflict pain, before the advent of anesthetization, was a primary character trait sought in a surgeon or dentist, suggesting that such an ability provided the power and authority for other ideological institutions as well:

> The practice of most professions in the eighteenth-century America was a harsh and grim business. Educators, from school masters to college presidents, plied the rattan and ferule. . . . Physicians bled, blistered, and purged, while dentists and surgeons performed their operations on screaming, struggling patients. The need to inflict great physical pain on clients pervaded daily professional life. It constituted an integral part of the self-image, ideology, and organization of most eighteenth-century professions.
>
> (242)

It also provided the muscle in the racket of controlling children. And though medical procedures rarely necessitate as much pain infliction as they did in previous centuries, the controllability of children is still exploited. It is not difficult to imagine Michael B. Rothenberg's admission from 1980 still applying in today's medical practice: "A lot of people go into pediatrics because they are more comfortable with children than they are with adults or because they have an urgent need to be in control of their patients" (23). Denial is a component of that ability and continued in the twentieth century perhaps as a means of appeasing doctor guilt or adult frustration. In fact, passionate denial seems to be a sign of a guilty conscience struggling with cognitive dissonance. In 1990, A. R. Lloyd-Thomas would argue,

> The concept that neonates do not feel pain was very convenient, in that pain relief could justifiably be withheld and the well-recognized dangers of giving powerful analgesics to these patients could therefore be circumvented. Indeed, this practice may be reinforced by physicians who routinely perform painful procedures and who reduce their own sympathetic distress by cognitive restructuring which is expressed as a disbelief in the subjective distress of the infant.
>
> (87)

The young, who play no part in legitimated discourses used to exploit their precarity and justify their mistreatment, are easily misrepresented in such "cognitive restructuring."

Denial of juvenile pain was sometimes absolute and unwavering. When Helen Neal was doing research for her 1978 book *The Politics of Pain*, she felt that no one wanted to discuss child pain in particular:

> It seemed that there was about this subject an unconscious conspiracy of denial. Among physicians this denial, more perhaps a disregard, was especially

marked. Neither callous nor cruel, their attitude was more a turning away from a situation they felt helpless to control.

(135)

Gary Walco et al. add that the insistence that "the pain is not that bad" may also be out of insecurity: "Our needs may also lead us to downplay a child's suffering to alleviate our own feelings of inadequacy" (2003, 158). Influenced by the medical norm, society at large tended to accept the denial of infant and even child pain:

> [A]s recently as the late 1980s and early 1990s, most people – and that includes many health-care practitioners – thought that infants either felt no pain, or did not remember it once it took place. . . . Thus, male infants were routinely circumcised without the use of pain medication, and because of concerns about giving anesthetics to infants, many babies underwent surgery without receiving painkillers.

> (Krane 249)

According to one study of child patients, researchers found no analgesics prescribed "despite diagnoses such as traumatic amputation of the foot, excision of a neck mass, and heminephrectomy" (Schechter et al. 1986, 11). Studies from the 1980s consistently indicated that the younger the patient, the less likely they would receive pain medication. David Morris describes one: "[A] study of Emergency Department records over a five month period in 1987–1988 showed that children with painful conditions were twice as likely as adults to receive no medication" (146). And even where suitable analgesics are prescribed, they are less likely to be actually given to juvenile patients: "[N]urses, the final common pathway for analgesic administration, tend to use less potent narcotics at lower doses if given a chance" (Schechter 1989, 789). This legacy far outlived any justifications. In 1996 Varsha Bhatt-Mehta would argue, "The pathophysiology of pain in children and adults is similar. This similarity suggests that the treatment of pain in children should be as aggressive as that in adults, regardless of the child's age" (761). Yet in 2003 Gary Walco et al. would still complain that "infants and young children often receive little attention to their pain and are forced to endure a great deal of untreated suffering" (157).

Some have indicated the increased narrowing into divided medical specializations as part of the problem. Mary S. Sheridan reports that a study from 1986 found that "[a]lthough 91 percent of surveyed pediatricians believed that children felt 'adultlike' pain by age two, only 77 percent of family practitioners and 59 percent of surgeons agreed" (92). Neil Schechter reports that

> when asked about situations outside of their common experience, physicians are able to look at pain problems more objectively and tend to be more liberal with analgesics, while within their purview, they tend to handle pain problems in the manner in which they were taught, which tends to be with less concern about pain.

> (1989, 789)

Tradition can create inertia and willful ignorance where the need to consider individual experience is concerned, especially where a paradigm shift is needed to
collectively recognize child pain.

In the late 1980s, due to the pervasive use of the procedure, male circumcision
became the issue that served as a rallying point for reform in the treatment of
infant, and by association child, pain. A procedure that is considered unnecessary
by most, it is still quite common and in some cases, still unanesthetized. Neil
Schechter writes,

> It is unfathomable that adults would be tied down and sutured or circumcised
> without appropriate sedation or analgesia, or that the pain following surgery
> would not be even considered in the orders written. Yet such is the case with
> children.
>
> (1989, 784)

Circumcision also provides an excellent example of how easily ideological motives
can be imposed in medical decisions for children and established as unquestion-
able tradition through history. The ideological motives for this imposition of pain
on nonconsenting infants are made even clearer when one considers earlier cam-
paigns for circumcision as a way of preventing masturbation. In 1935, the misfor-
tunately named R. W. Cockshut[6] explicitly advocated,

> I suggest that all male children should be circumcised. . . . Civilization . . .
> requires chastity, and the glans of the circumcised rapidly assumes a leathery
> texture less sensitive than skin. Thus the adolescent has his attention drawn
> to his penis much less often.
>
> (quoted in Fox 170)

Moral prejudice, not concern for the child's body, made the procedure so prevalent.

Marie Fox and Michael Thomson would write in 2005 that "[o]nly limited consideration is given to the seemingly obvious fact that circumcision is the excision
of healthy tissue from a child unable to give his consent for no demonstrable
medical benefit" (170). So, basically, in the twenty-first century two scholars argue
that the nineteenth-century method of relying on infants' manageability is still
used to justify the "mute infant" as an "ideal medical subject." Fox and Thomson
conclude that doctors continue to take "advantage of the fact that performing the
procedure on neonates who were incapable of resisting made it considerably easier
to practice" (175). Not only is the unnecessary procedure imposed on newborns
(when they are incapable of informed consent) with the possible depletion of their
sexual pleasure in later life, but the exposure to pain, especially if unanesthetized
with postoperative pain untreated, can contribute to pain in later life. Walco et al.
argue, "Analyses showed greater pain responses across the board in boys who were
circumcised without local anesthetic in contrast to those who were uncircumcised"
(2003, 161). This raises another concern about long-term effects of undertreating
infant and child pain—far from being easily forgotten, the body remembers pain,[7]

and current studies of chronic neuropathic pain indicate that one of its causes is early untreated pain.

But concern for later pain problems won't convince those who hold onto an outdated denial of child pain, which has been historically powerful. In 1978, one doctor told Helen Neal, "Children don't have chronic pain. They either quickly recover or they die" (139). Some used the theory that myelination of nerves continues to develop into childhood as reassurance that pain response in younger patients was less intense than in adults. But it is now understood that infant pain is very real: "We now know that babies feel pain. In fact, experts in fetal development believe that the nerve pathways in a twenty-nine-week-old fetus are functional and capable of transmitting pain signals from the body to the brain" (Krane 2005, 249–250). Not only is their pain greater than once thought, but if left untreated it can lead to more pain in later life. Lonnie K. Zeltzer explains that

> [m]edical thinking did not begin to change until the late 1980s after several studies were published in scientific journals showing that even the youngest children – premature babies – experience pain. In fact, babies may be more sensitive to pain because the parts of their nervous system that control pain are not fully developed. We also know that significant early pain experiences can actually have a big effect on the developing nervous system, cause children to become more sensitive to pain, and may contribute to the development of chronic pain in later life.
>
> (2)

Leora Kuttner further explains,

> Although pain messages are conducted more slowly in newborn babies, these messages have a shorter distance to travel. Moreover, because they do not have the ability to modulate the transmission of pain signals . . . [they] persist in the infants' systems, and painful procedures produce a much stronger physiological response in an infant than in an adolescent or adult.
>
> (26)

Quite contrary to pervasive historic ideologies in public discourse, infants experience pain more intensely than older patients,[8] and this translates into memorable pain. Frederic A. Berry and George A. Gregory concluded as early as 1987 that premature neonates may have residual trace memories of operative pain (291). Pain in early childhood can create ready nerve pathways that enable future communication of pain within the body, whether or not there is an actual external stimulus:[9] "[T]hus, early, untreated pain experiences appear to sensitize the child to subsequent painful experiences" (Walco et al. 2003, 161). Early pain stimuli do not give us a higher tolerance for later pain—they train our brain to quicken and sharpen the pain response.

Looking back from the first quarter of the twenty-first century it is clear that for children, the "Age of Pain" did not stop in the nineteenth but continued throughout most of the next century. Even though "[b]y 1995, there was almost universal agreement that newborns and neonates perceived pain," according to a 1996 survey, "[d]rugs were reported to be used infrequently even for the most painful procedures" in infants, including circumcision, insertion of chest and gavage tubes, umbilical catheterization, arterial or venous cutdown, lumbar punctures, intramuscular injections, intravenous lines, and tracheal suctioning (McGrath and Unruh 2002, 558–560). In 2005 Lonnie Zeltzer would report that "[e]very year, 1.5 million U.S. children have surgery, and many of them have inadequate pain relief. For about 20%, the pain becomes chronic" (4). Elliott Krane writes that infants' pain "is believed to have a significant, perhaps even life-long impact on them," resulting in later learning delays, chronic pain, and increased sensitivity to painful stimuli (250). Of child pain he writes, "

> [C]hronic pain experienced during childhood may predispose individuals to more debilitating pain later in life; in other words, pain begets pain. This is because chronic pain changes the way the central nervous system processes and transmits pain nerve signals, making it sensitive to stimulation over time.
>
> (18)

Flor Herta and Niels Birbaumer argue that "chronification" is a "learnt conditioned response" through the development of "cortical pain memories" (119–120). Tess Burton explains that

> [p]ersistent pain can produce a cycle of chemical and electrical action and reaction in the body that initiates an automatic feedback loop, in which the nervous system begins to generate pain on its own, resulting in 'neuropathic pain' for which there is no external cause.
>
> (26)

Pain continues to be undertreated for people of all ages, but especially so for children, in spite of these risks.

McGrath and Unruh argue that "there are safe and effective pharmacologic methods to control pain from the most painful procedures such as circumcision and chest tube insertion but they are not universally used" (560). In fact, even "[c]omfort measures such as the use of pacifiers and bundling are not universally used" (560). And fear of addiction is overstated in popular discourse. Though patients can become tolerant and even dependent, which is true for many medications (including corticosteroids, asthma inhalers, and insulin), these outcomes are easily dealt with through managed tapering off according to doctor's instructions, especially for patients young enough to be dependent upon others for dispensation. Elliot Krane reports that addiction is a low risk in children: only "5 percent of the American population have the genetic basis for becoming addicted given the right social circumstances"—circumstances associated with adolescence and adulthood, not childhood (175). Neil Schechter writes, "The available studies suggest that addiction is extraordinarily rare after hospital-based use of narcotics for acute pain problems. . . . To withhold adequate pain relief from a suffering patient on the theoretical grounds of addiction potential is not only inhumane, but incorrect" (1989, 787). And it persists in the highest drug-consuming country in the world at the height of pill culture.

Of course any drug with risks of addiction or accidental overdose (which is on the rise in adult patients) is impractical for daily use or for a chronic condition. My point in addressing such drugs is to indicate the depth of hypocrisy in adult-serving discourses. The bias against narcotics due to fears of addicting children seems particularly overstated in light of unheeded warnings of a much greater risk for addiction from widely prescribed non-narcotic medications in the pediatric population. Nadine Lambert, professor of educational psychology, presented findings at the 1998 National Institute of Health Consensus Conference on ADHD that Ritalin

> might contribute to later drug abuse. Her study of 400 children with ADHD showed that by the time children treated with Ritalin reached their mid-twenties, they had double the rates of cocaine abuse and cigarette smoking as young adults who hadn't taken Ritalin in childhood.
>
> (Diller 94)

Exacerbating this potential risk is that stimulants are being taken for longer periods of a young person's life:

> Whereas virtually all children taking stimulants in the 1970s and 1980s stopped taking them at around age thirteen, when hyperactivity tends to fade on its own, current standards of care mandate that many adolescents continue to take these meds through high school and even into college.
>
> (Diller 98)

Risks for addictive behaviors, and exposure to probable triggers of addiction, begin to be more of a factor in adolescence and young adulthood.

We can no longer assume that undertreatment of child pain in the United States stems from legitimate protective fears of drugging children. The reality seems to be that we don't mind drugging kids at all, if it keeps them in control. Letty Coltin Pogrebin predicted this reality in her observation that "[a]s a society, we love children when they are under control. . . . [C]hildren are the last remaining subjects of domination" (47). If the real agenda is simply controlling children, treating child pain becomes unnecessary. A child in pain is easily controlled (that's one reason pain is the primary mechanism of torture—it is brutally disempowering[10]). The seemingly contradictory mandate of protecting kids from drugs, except in the form of behavior-modifying pills dispensed by the school nurse, took on a particularly absurd pitch at the beginning of the twenty-first century, where adult control over child agency was the obvious priority. At its most perverse, perhaps, in the zero-tolerance policies that emerged all over the country during this era of authoritarian education was the 2003 strip search of Savana Redding, then 13, for two 200 mg Ibuprofen tablets (yes, over-the-counter drugs commonly taken by teenage girls for menstrual cramps,[11] in either 400 mg doses or prescription 800 mg, neither of which Savana even had). Migraineur Caleb Hood complains that under zero-tolerance policy the maximum amount of ibuprofen he could carry in school, after much discussion and annually repeated documentation from his doctor (who actually prescribed it in 600 mg pills), was 400 mg. That this is absurd is only part of the point—the larger one is that such policy keeps children in pain for simply not fitting a bureaucratic rule that fails to take child pain into account.

During the time Savana Redding was in middle school there were many highly publicized national stories about school staff stealing and selling student prescription drugs: "School nurses, 'teachers of the year,' and principals are among those found 'liberating' Ritalin from school coffers" (Toby Miller 152; see also Mayes 148). Nevertheless, fruitless efforts to catch students dealing drugs continued, and some have been carried out through rights-violating undercover entrapment rings, like those carried out at Paloma Valley High School and Perris High School in 2013. I need not dwell on the neglectful hypocrisy encouraged by this era of zero tolerance but have to note the irony of violating one child's rights over suspected possession of over-the-counter pain medication while lining up many of her classmates to get their dose of street-valued speed from an adult to keep them manageable.

The school of pain

Shulamith Firestone writes, "If childhood was only an abstract concept, then the modern school was the institution that built it into a reality" (92). The building of the current edu-pharmaceutical complex that creates controllable students can be traced back through the centuries. The ideologies that built it are pervasive in public discourse, including popular children's books. In Susan Coolidge's (1872) novel *What Katy Did*, the title character is injured in a fall and paralyzed as a result. Katy's "invalid" cousin Helen comes to visit and shore her up, providing an explicitly didactic model of coping behavior. Katy asks the saintly Helen, "How do you manage to be so sweet and beautiful and patient when you're feeling badly all the time, and can't do anything, or walk, or stand?" (132). Helen shares her own wisdom on how to appropriately suffer by inviting Katy to commit herself to "the School of Pain" (133). In her own room and bed, she is to study:

> Well, there's the lesson of Patience. That's one of the hardest studies. You can't learn much of it at a time, but every bit you get by heart makes the next bit easier. And there's the lesson of Cheerfulness. And the lesson of Making the Best of Things.
>
> (134)

Helen's advice reminds us that a great part of healing before the twentieth century, and still for some conditions, depends upon waiting. "Patient" denotes a sufferer but also someone who suffers patiently in order to heal, or (a bit more cynically) to be as little a burden as possible on others who must take responsibility for one's care. Coolidge's novel doesn't just teach girls how to be passively silent young ladies; it teaches children how to be passively silent patients and students. Jenny Slater has pointed out that "[t]he message around disability we are delivered from [such] texts is that one cannot be both 'grownup' and 'disabled'; disability is equated with a childlike way of being" (45). And the good "disabled" child does not complain. Echoing the doctor cited above who claimed that children "either quickly recover or they die" (Neal 139), the cultural message here is "get better or disappear." From such a perspective, there is simply no acknowledgment of diverse possibilities for children living well with impairments (however variously defined). Such a social space is made to seem irreversibly liminal, invisible, cast out of the social whole.

Helen's advice also suggests the power of pain to subdue and force children to adapt and conform to societal expectations, as well as reminding that teaching how to do this is one goal of schools. Often, the ideologies used to control children are far more subtle than the religious instruction and pain that teach Katy, but Helen's analogy of becoming a good patient with being a good student indicates the ideological similarities between the institutions of medicine and education, which are still two of the most powerful ideological state apparatuses in a child's socialization.

The common motive of controlling children explains why throughout the emergence, coexistence, and even dominance of completely conflicting ideologies about how to treat children, adults are so incapable of seeing their hypocrisies clearly. Medical and pedagogical control reinforced a deeper, unquestioned prejudice. Martin Pernick sees emerging philosophies about pain and children from the nineteenth century as related to evolving pedagogies at the time: "The introduction of surgical anesthesia bears close comparison with the decline of other painful therapies in medicine and with the loosening use of whipping in education and criminal justice" (8). The means of controlling children in schools would become more bureaucratic, and misguidedly normative:

> From a twentieth-century viewpoint, the nineteenth-century creation of large, age-graded, ability-tracked, factory-styled school systems seems the height of impersonal bureaucracy. But to antebellum educators, preoccupied with replacing the undifferentiated one-room school, the particularization possible in a finely graded bureaucracy seemed to be a move toward greater recognition of pupil individuality. Teachers, like doctors, confused the recognition of diversity with the recognition of individuality.
>
> (146–147)

Within the complicated legacy of pedagogy in the United States, then, are the contradictory aims of privileging diversification yet relying on heavy norming, which effectively discourages and obscures difference. James E. Block has argued that this paradox is at the crux of American citizenship, which, influenced by John Locke, "redefined the path to voluntary adult membership by locating it in the controllable confines of childhood" (19). Smoothing over the contradiction between its commitments, "Americans thus demanded of child rearing a seemingly paradoxical outcome: an individual both convinced that he was entirely self-determining and yet fully adaptive in his conduct" (21). Pernick's and Block's insights relate significantly to today's politics of youth and disability. The legacy of American individualism is paired with an extreme reliance on norming, the contradiction between which is constantly elided through ideologies that dominate in schools and medical practice. If we acknowledge that such a fundamental contradiction lies at the heart of unquestioned health and educational ideologies, it may be easier to tease out explanations of how (too) easily these ideologies have failed to recognize and serve the special needs of impaired individuals.

One clear example of the contradictory challenge contemporary educators and students must negotiate can be seen in the near impossibility of reconciling the progress of the Individuals with Disabilities Education Act (IDEA) with the agenda of the No Child Left Behind Act (NCLB) of 2001. On one hand, mainstreaming students with disabilities into inclusive public schools was a long-needed improvement in terms of reducing discrimination and opening educational opportunities. Judith Warner echoes a common sentiment: "Unable to attend public school, severely learning-disabled or autistic children in the past became invisible. Now, they are seen" (47). But with the increased pressure for "accountability" among schools, teachers, and students that resulted from NCLB, or, as Edward Bloor satirically dubs it, "Leave No High-Scoring Child Behind" (61), administrators sometimes (illegally) discourage the enrollment of learning-disabled students in their schools, find loopholes justifying their exclusion, or explicitly abuse them. Sharon Lynn Nichols adds,

> Districts can allow students with severe cognitive challenges to take a special version of the test, but only if these students constitute 1 percent or less of the student body. . . . Not surprisingly, any school with a special-education population over 1 percent is likely to show less annual progress than other schools. Thus, special-education students are punished when they cannot pass the regular version of the test.
>
> (65)

Critics of NCLB, like Barbara Bennett Woodhouse, argue that "[e]quality for children must mean something other than identical treatment," indicating how incompatible high-stakes testing is with individualized instruction. The era of standardization has had a disastrous effect in the limitations placed on effectively mainstreaming students with disabilities whose unique differences and special pedagogical needs are deprioritized in favor of imposing conformity with a norm of developmental pace. In recent years, schools report shocking statistics of students (sometimes as high as 50%) failing the third grade because of standardized reading test scores. In spite of the IDEA, problems of mainstreaming disabled students into the climate of NCLB, zero-tolerance policy, and Race to the Top reveal that competitive assessment models normatize, lump together, and stigmatize slower-paced or differently abled learners with increased standardization, increasing the drugging of students for performance rather than fostering their health, individualized abilities, and self-sufficiency through less testing and greater flex time.

Increased pressure to perform in the classroom has surely increased student stress, especially for those who are learning or improving in different skills at different paces. With increased accountability the expected pace has increased considerably. Lawrence Diller observes,

> The demands on children's educational performance and behavior in school have vastly increased over the past twenty-five years. I shake my head in uneasy wonderment when I compare what pediatricians considered 'normal' development for a five-year-old in 1980 with pediatricians' performance expectations for five-year-olds today. Before 1990 I was satisfied with a child's intellectual growth. . . . [I]f at age five the child spoke clearly and used and understood oral language like other children his age. But then I became aware of a downward push, coming down from the high schools through the middle and grade schools and affecting the goals of early education. So by the early 1990s, five-year-olds were expected to decode letters and sounds, write and spell simple words, and perform simple addition and subtraction.
>
> (10)

While the general public bemoans the poor state of American education in the global context, standards, not student performances, rise. And these standards become an artificially inflated, imposed new norm,

> Although many children are capable of handling the more difficult curriculum, a large minority cannot. . . . Twenty years ago, most of these kids would have been considered developmentally normal.[12] Now they are diagnosed with learning disorders because they cannot meet the new standards.
>
> (11)

Judith Warner, who wrote a nuanced counterargument to media concerns about overmedicated children, agrees with Diller on this point:

> Kindergarteners are now expected to know how to read, have mastered some basic math facts, and to be able to write simple sentences by the time they graduate to first grade. In some districts, kindergarteners are required to do as much as two hours of daily reading drills. . . . Reading instruction came to stress speed and a narrow definition of proficiency, with the result that other aspects of reading for pleasure, or for deeper meaning, were sacrificed. By March 2006, 71 percent of the nation's school districts had reduced time for history, music, and other subjects in favor of more time for testable reading and math.
>
> (181)

Focusing attention solely on quantifiable aspects of learning is a ridiculous over-simplification of the learning process, not to mention that we all have different processes and paces, and need to be free to advance in unmeasurable ways. Educators all over the country have contested or bent to the pressure to teach to tests. The school principal in Edward Bloor's satire on standardization, *Story Time*, reasons, "If information is not tested in any of the fifty United States, is there any reason for a United States student to learn it?" (103–104). But the problem isn't just the narrowing curriculum and stressful testing; it is the failure to understand the role of assessment in education, and a failure to understand that norms are mathematical constructs, which instead are now taken as essential, permanent indicators of success that in turn discourage recognition of individualized learning.

The connection between increased pressures to succeed on tests and the increase of prescribed performance-enhancing drugs is more than simply correlative. Stephen Hinshaw found a direct causal relationship between states which adopted NCLB and increasing diagnoses of ADHD: "In 2007, 15.6 percent of kids between the ages of 4 and 17 in North Carolina had at some point received an ADHD diagnosis. In California, that number was 6.2 percent" (Koerth-Baker). Eliminating race and income as factors, Hinshaw found that

> kids in North Carolina were nearly twice as likely to be given diagnoses of ADHD as those in California. . . . Nothing seemed to explain the difference – until he looked at educational policies. . . . North Carolina was one of the first to adopt such a program; California was one of the last; . . . [H]e found that when a state passed laws punishing or rewarding schools for their standardized test scores, *ADHD diagnosis increased by 22 percent in the first four years after No Child Left Behind was implemented.*
>
> (Koerth-Baker, my emp)

Lawrence Diller also recounts the interconnectedness of test pressures and seeking pharmaceutical advantage: "[I]n recent years I've noticed a mini-uptick in the number of calls I receive about a month or two before the Scholastic Aptitude Test (SAT) is administered" (37). Though such examples have been exaggerated in the media, the direct causal relationship between authoritarian, assessment-crazed policy and our selective willingness to drug children is telling.

Toby Miller writes that high-stakes testing creates "incentives to define pupils as disabled, via special-education programs that support low-income parents and schools once children are diagnosed with ADHD" (147). A successful means of getting appropriate tutoring to some of the students who need it, such diagnoses also have a downside—often a prescription alone is administered, as a quick fix: "We already substitute medication for nondrug services at school" (Diller 61). If students successfully get greater aid without or with drugs, that's fine, but being pressured to perform just for the numbers game is inexcusable. Alfie Kohn gets to the heart of the problem: "Setting children against one another in contests, so that one can't succeed unless others fail, has demonstrably negative effects—on psychological health, relationships, intrinsic motivation and achievement—for winners and losers alike" (61). Ultimately we are twisting children's priorities if all they learn at school is that success lies in scores, and that performance drugs and scores bring funding and security, two things, apparently, more important to the nation than children's health.

We are stressing kids out over something relatively meaningless: grades. Alfie Kohn writes,

> The available research suggests that there are three predictable effects when students are led to focus on bringing home better report cards: They tend to become less interested in the learning itself, to think in a more superficial fashion, and to prefer the easiest possible task.
>
> (138)

On a theoretical level such motives and pressures also miss the point. Programs that require constant "growth" or that students "race to the top" seem to be as oblivious to math as they fear their students are. Deborah Meier explains:

> Demanding that more kids get higher scores on standardized tests – be they IQ tests or achievement tests – is, under these circumstances, something like demanding that students line up faster so that more will be in the front half of the line. Even seemingly modest demands, that all high school graduates read 'at least on a tenth grade level,' are statistically nonsense.
>
> (103)

In a culture that treats norms as essential truths, ironically, many young students have no sense of how norms are created. I was shocked during one of my upper-level college classes, in which we were discussing some cases Lawrence Diller describes[13] of students (and parents) who are unhappy with getting B and C grades, for whom that was enough to justify medication. One of my students, an education major, asked, "Shouldn't everyone be above average?" I was floored. My students didn't know what a bell curve was, or that Cs are supposed to represent the average, or that average, in and of itself, is a perfectly legitimate place to be. I'm not sure which of those realizations made me sadder. If one accepts grading as a necessary practice (I personally find it useless, but it's part of my job), then one should at least comprehend the hierarchy it creates and how it is created. Lennard Davis contextualizes the bell-curve legacy as a result of "the hegemony of the middle," by which averages become "paradoxically a kind of ideal, a position to be devoutly wished" (2013, 2). When we essentialize averages we are capable of such mathematically nonsensical concepts of "raising" them, which can never be an equitable practice because "equality is therefore based not on an ethical notion but on a quasi-scientific one" (Davis 2002, 105). Norms are mathematical constructs that have become utilized as diagnostic tools, but we must be educated and self-aware of how to use them rather than granting them such deterministic power. This would help all students, not just young migraineurs for whom tests can be a trigger, and who are also more likely to struggle with school experience.

Norms are not simply abusive because they are foolishly and stringently applied. They also encourage generalizing and dismissal, which only benefits the "average" majority. The same essentializing confusion dominates our attitudes toward health. The hegemony of a narrowly defined ability rests on normative notions of health that hide their own relativism, which Georges Canguilhem, among others, has pointed to as a damaging ideal:

> As if perfect health were not a normative concept, an ideal type? Strictly speaking a norm does not exist,[14] it plays its role which is to devalue existence by allowing its correction. To say that perfect health does not exist is simply saying that the concept of health is not one of an existence, but of a norm whose function and value is to be brought into contact with existence in order to stimulate modification.
>
> (77)

Perfect students, normal students, even average students do not exist. These are simply constructs used to define children within the institutional ideologies of their schools. Likewise, there is no essential healthy child or ability, and those who become diagnosed with disease or dubbed as disabled are being presented with identities that should not be used just to fit and "correct" them toward a mathematical norm—they are meant to ensure diverse accommodations. We need to think beyond norms by listening to individuals' developing needs—no matter how fluctuating and invisible their reasons may be. And we can value the existence of the differing minds and bodies of children.

Rather than overtesting, selectively drugging, and casting out "unhealthy" impaired children, our social institutions have to be able to recognize and support individualized modes of thriving. For example, C. M. Shifflett views migraineurs as a potential vanguard in detecting structural problems: "In many modern money mines and cube farms, migraineurs are the canaries, a first alert of Sick Building Syndrome before more subtle signs of fatigue, dizziness, ill health, and increasing absenteeism are recognized by other employees" (9). Child migraineurs have heightened sensory responses that could help others to consider that the standard American diet shouldn't be the standard, school lunches should be accordingly reformed, schools shouldn't be testing factories, and school nurses should be allowed to practice healing, not reduced to serving as dispensaries. Offering children with migraine a quiet, private cot in a small dark room when needed wouldn't hurt either.

In the historic neglect of pediatric pain and the current trend of medicating child behaviors instead, the common premise is the desirability of a controllable child. Hopefully we can fight the prejudicial power of silencing ideologies by exposing the undeniable physical and emotional toll they take on child bodies. Some have responded with empathy and empowered agency, and history is replete with strategies for counterattacking both pain and social forces silencing those in it. Exploring literary expressions as well as contrasting realities will be one of the aims of my next chapter. Part of showing the material reality of individual experiences will also involve a look at the numerous stereotypes rigidly set in public views through literary and popular culture. Though they might make migraine appear to be more concrete to the general public, they require debunking to effect a more accurate and diversified visibility.

Notes

1 For example, "GlaxoSmithKline, the biggest pharmaceutical company, settled charges for 3 billion dollars in the United States for illegal marketing of dangerous antidepressant drugs to children that made them suicidal and that had not been approved by safety regulators" (Spronk 190).
2 Analogous groupings of young humans with nonhuman animals has been used injuriously (Peter Singer) and proactively (Ruth O'Brien). I will play up the positive possibilities more as my argument progresses in later chapters.
3 Such stories might be contrasted with more recent struggles between parents who refuse to drug their children for ADHD and their school districts. In some of the worst abuses, parents have been given ultimatums to medicate their child or face his or her expulsion:

> Public school administrators, long enthusiastic adherents to a "just say no" policy on drug use, have a new motto for the parents of certain tiny soldiers in the war on drugs: Medicate or else! It is a new and troubling twist in the psychiatric drugs saga, in which public schools have begun to issue ultimatums to parents of hard-to-handle kids, saying they will not allow students to attend conventional classes unless they are medicated. In the most extreme cases, parents unwilling to give their kids drugs are being reported by their schools to local offices of child protective services, the implication being that by withholding drugs, the parents are guilty of neglect.
>
> (Diller, 51)

Some parents have even been threatened with losing child custody (54). This scenario became so prevalent that several states legislated against the practice: "In July of 2001, Minnesota became the first state to bar schools and child protection agencies from telling parents they must put their children on drugs to treat disorders like attention deficit hyperactivity disorder" (Zernike and Petersen). Connecticut bars "any school or staff member from discussing drug treatments with a parent" (Zernike and Petersen). Ironically, in my state many parents lose temporary or even permanent custody of their children due to methamphetamine habits, only for their children to be taken into foster care and put on legally enforced prescriptions of amphetamines.
4 Dorothea Z. Lack writes that "physicians believe the pain of women to be psychological in origin more often than the pain of men" (63). Much has been written of the tendency to view women's complaints as neurotic or hysterical, which of course applies in the case of headaches as well: "Dr. Oliver Wendell Holmes marveled, 'She is so much more fertile in capacities of suffering than a man. She has so many varieties of headache'" (Pernick 149).
5 The original source adds this information on the patient: "an impatient boy, tired of a six months' confinement to bed" (Dupierris 294).
6 Seriously, real name; I checked the original source thinking it must be a practical joke. Cited from *British Medical Journal* (Oct. 19, 1935): 763–764.
7 The body also remembers in the form of phobias. Consider the example of Rod, who was born in 1964 prematurely and spent four months in an incubator getting painful procedures (when they were regularly done with no pain control). His medical trauma resulted in a debilitating fear of needles: he "cannot stay in a room where there's a needle," he says. "I feel like such a wimp. I can face and wrestle an armed man to the ground. But when a pint-sized nurse comes toward me with a needle, I clear out of the room! It's crazy!" (Kuttner, 23). Likewise, birth trauma has been connected with the development of claustrophobia, which feels not like fear at all but a rationally

uncontrollable fight-or-flight instinct. Mary S Sheridan writes, "According to family reports, some seem to carry memories of difficult hospitalizations for a long time. Others seem to have permanently increased tolerances for pain." However, "the great degree of learning about infants' pain leaves the field open to speculation and the speculation open to the needs of the theorist" (86).

8 Here's a slightly more specialized explanation:

> Although early research emphasizing incomplete myelination implied that children responded differently to noxious stimulation and questioned whether they experienced pain, most recent data using spectrographic analysis of infant cries, physiologic responses to circumcision, and standardized behavioral observation of children undergoing medical procedures all report that infants and young children clearly experience discomfort. In fact, Haslam, using laboratory-induced pain, found that younger children had a lower threshold for pain than older children. Similarly, Jay et al. found that children's distress during medical procedures was inversely proportional to their age.
>
> (Schechter 1986, 14)

9 Or, in medical jargon, "in the neonatal period, peripheral nerve networks are going through a process of increasing differentiation. When repeatedly insulted with painful stimuli, this process is altered such that lower levels of stimulation potentiate relatively significant nociceptive responses" (Walco et al. 2003, 161).

10 Political manipulation through pain is not limited to torture. There is evidence to suggest that the United States actively engaged in the withholding pain relief as a means of building political power and even biological warfare in World War II. According to drug-war scholar, William Avilés, "During the 1930s and 1940s the United States sought to stockpile and control the world's market for opium and coca leaves as well as their manufactured outputs (heroin, morphine and cocaine) . . . to deprive the Axis powers from getting access to these essential war-time drugs" (personal email). Ironically the block on German access to essential pain-killing supplies necessitated and so instigated German innovations and rise to greater economic power in this market. For more details see McAllister (2000, 145–148) and Reiss (2014, 28–29).

11 Regina Dengler and Heather Roberts studied reported use of over-the-counter painkillers by adolescents and found "[g]irls aged 14–15 are more likely than others to have used at least one of the drugs in the previous week, with 40 percent of girls in this age group having used a non-prescribed painkiller" (437).

12 I'd be remiss if I didn't mention that part of this shift is also a result of racial politics. Christine E. Sleeter exposed, as early as the 1980s, that the category of *learning disabled* "was created by white middle class parents in an effort to differentiate their children from low-achieving low-income and minority children. . . . [I]t upheld their intellectual normalcy and the normalcy of their home backgrounds" as well as granting already privileged children more services to help them compete with others (210). Judith Warner's account shows that these inequities are still very much at play.

13 Most notable is the case of an eight-year-old: "Ned seemed pretty miserable over his C grades. . . . His parents and the school expected so much more from Ned. It didn't help that both his parents had finished graduate school, and Ned's IQ had tested at about 130. Ned's mood in my office ranged from thoughtful to depressingly somber and reflected the collective disappointment over his performance" (4). Essentializing him based on his IQ score is bad enough, but the solution agreed upon by therapist, parents, and teacher? To begin a rewards system. And the punishment used for negative reinforcement? Cutting his time from reading – something he did much of for pleasure, and needless to say, is of educational value, just not the kind they were measuring at his school (6).

14 Canguilhem admits this as a "facile relativism," but it is usefully articulated (77). Lennard Davis expounds a similar argument in the context of disability: "Under normalcy, no one is or can be normal, just as no one is or can be equal. All have to work hard to make it seem that they conform, and so the person with disabilities is singled out as a dramatic case of not belonging. This identification makes it easier for the rest to think they fit the paradigm" (2002, 105).

3 Materia medica and literary migraine

> I begin to assemble what weapons I can find
> Because sometimes to stay alive you got to kill your mind
>
> Twenty One Pilots, "Migraine"[1]

Whereas pain has been selectively ignored in children, migraine has been culturally dismissed to varying degrees in persons of all ages. N. Ann Davis argues that persons living with invisible impairments are socially required to prove their special needs through confessional narratives. Joanna Kempner shows that though migraine has been known and treated for at least 6,000 years, it is still a socially "contested illness" with a "legitimacy deficit" (12, 9). Part of the problem, as Susannah B. Mintz explains, is that "headache is both one of the most common forms of chronic pain and one of the most clichéd" (2014, 84–85). Early terms such as "megrim" or "the megrims" were commonly synonymous with "low spirits" or even a "whim" or "fancy" (*Oxford English Dictionary*). As a socially dismissed and medically liminal experience, migraine requires extensive narratives to convince others of its existence. Yet, authentic versions of these narratives rarely make it beyond blogs and the self-help sections of bookstores. Migraineurs are almost as hard to find, identified precisely, in literary and popular culture as child migraineurs are in major migraine studies. Sure, they exist, but at a tiny fraction of the frequencies with which they exist in the everyday lives of real individuals. Where represented, however, literary migraine carries an ongoing record of treatments and revealing prejudices. Joanna Kempner writes that "disease categories reflect the specific historical and social contexts in which they are created. Disease entities are as social as they are biological" (10). My analysis will provide historical contextualization of both the social and biological beliefs that have shaped literary migraine, with an eye to explaining why children are once again underrepresented and too easily overlooked.

In this chapter I will demonstrate how the compulsive narratives of literary and material history serve to silence or legitimate migraine, through analysis of literary tropes, metaphors, character stereotypes, compensatory outings, diagnostic criticism, gendered and ageist medicalization, medical interventions, and coping strategies. By using literary and filmic examples, I hope to demonstrate social attitudes toward migraine, girding each with a materializing context from both medical history and intimate bodily interventions. Migraine plays a complicated role especially in breaking mind-body binarisms, which it both phenomenologically affirms and medically dismantles. These discourses also reveal that child pain is silenced and invisible in fiction as well, if represented at all, but I will promote bringing it out of obscurity to encourage legitimating visibility.

"Killing" the mind

Migraineurs have been assembling weapons against their pain throughout history, but understanding how they have been used requires some nuance along with bare facts. In the opening scenes of the film *That Beautiful Somewhere* (2006), its protagonist, an archeologist named Catherine, has a migraine attack triggered by the lighting as she gives a public lecture. We see her struggle later in full-attack mode, moaning like an animal,[2] shedding tears but holding back sobs in her efforts to be still. It's a fantastic and rare rendering of a migraine attack, capped off with a stunning transition. As she cradles a drill in her hand and rocks on the edge of a bed, one can see not fear but desperate resolve, a far more dramatic version of the hesitance I felt the first time I injected myself with sumatriptan (a powerful halting sensation probably familiar to anyone the first time they inject themselves)— battling the skittish protective instinct, suddenly aware of the body's own powerful resistance to potential harm, then overriding it with the will of the mind. At that moment you have to treat your body as an other. Human medicine over animal body, reason over self-eclipsing pain. But what the film shows next is something much more sensational and affective. Catherine presses the drill to her temple, debates another moment, and presses it on. A split second shows the large drill bit start to turn, with a momentary auditory overlap—the undeniable high-pitched, power-tool whir, then an almost instantaneous cut to the next scene.

Over the years I've had the opportunity to describe this scene to many people. Most wince at the thought and then prepare a polite pitying expression on their faces. But if the film comes up during interviews with migraineurs, I've not once seen a wince in reaction. Instead appreciative nods beat me to the moment in which we imagine Catherine has trepanned her own skull, echoed with practical approval: "of course," "good idea," an only slightly hyperbolically intended "been there!" or even a comic "what sort of drill bit would you use? Masonry, perhaps." The film offers more than drama; it's affirmation. No blood, no gore, just the twisted glory of mind over matter (or is it matter over mind?). One blogger, Susan Jillian, responded to the film by pointing out, "What is cathartic is knowing someone cared enough to show it as it really is for those of us who have an extreme variation of the disease," and one of her commenters wrote that he "identified with the scene where the heroine took the drill with the 3/8 inch bit and placed it on her temple. I usually visualize using an ice pick myself . . ." (Jillian). In this type of imaginative coping, the migraineur projects the self outside of the body, taking hold of the weapon to enact control and procure relief. In such moments, migraine can blur the otherwise seemingly stark distinction between self-violence and self-preservation.

"Killing the mind" becomes a recurring trope of transcendent selfhood that legitimates migraineur experience and agency, though often seeming to regress into mind-body dualism.

The woman with the drill in the opening moment of *That Beautiful Somewhere* is at war with her body. And many migraineurs play out a similar battle in their minds, which can shift priorities profoundly. Thomas Jefferson learned from chronic headaches that "[t]he art of life is the avoiding of pain" (quoted in Friedman 664). Migraineur Virginia Woolf wrote that "literature does its best to maintain that its concern is with the mind; that the body is a sheet of glass through which the soul looks straight and clear" (317). When mind and body are at such odds, the artificiality of this device is quite apparent, and the "glass" through which we see ourselves is completely clouded, so that we cannot help but be aware of the body during "[t]hose great wars which it wages by itself, with the mind a slave to it" (318). When the body is under the duress of pain, the mind cannot engage in denials of vulnerability or idealizations of mental wholeness, clarity, and control. Instead, the mind seeks transcendence by acting out, sometimes violently, against the body. The now-common term "painkiller"[3] echoes this presumption of necessary violence—one might consider, in telling contrast, the "quieting powder" the child character Pollyanna is given, mentioned in the previous chapter (Porter 186). And people in pain are capable of the ultimate self-violence—suicide. Studies of the effects of prohibiting access to narcotics, like the opium and heroin previously available in the late nineteenth and early twentieth centuries, include revealing accounts of desperate migraineurs. Thomas Dormandy reports, "The wife of the local pastor in Bielefeld, not far from the Bayer [former mass producer of over-the-counter heroin] establishment, who had been denied continued injections against her attacks of migraine, committed suicide" (197). Addiction, in light of such cases, may be seen as a sometimes fatally complicating factor, but generally lesser evil, resulting from severe or chronic headaches and dependency on opiates. In a 1907 "Clinical History of Three Interesting Cases of Morphinism," a Dr. McKay includes an account of a 26-year old woman who "gave a history of nervous headaches since early childhood" (466). In 1918, Dr. Carl Scheffel would find that "insomnia and various types of recurrent headache rank foremost in the list of etiological factors" leading to drug addictions (853). David Courtwright et al. collected fascinating testimonies from narcotics addicts, many of whom became addicted due to inadequate palliative alternatives, which forced them to access pain relief illegally once opiates became legally regulated.[4] One, a migraineur they call Sam, describes his experience in the 1940s being "tossed around from doctor to doctor," none of whom were able to help: "I threatened suicide. I told him and the others that, if they couldn't cure me, I was going to kill myself. I was quite serious. I could no longer stand this pain" (72–73). Naomi Breslau et al. "found a greater than 4-fold[5] risk of suicide attempt in persons with migraine headaches, relative to controls who have never experienced headaches above mild intensity" (729). And risk of suicide significantly increases with severity of pain (723, 729). In light of these facts, trepanation might not seem so hard to believe.

In fact, trepanation is actually quite intuitive. Locate and counterattack the enemy, or as Billie Joe Armstrong sings, "drain the pressure from the swelling." Though trepanation is often thought of as a primitive form of punishment or sacrifice, historical evidence speaks to its existing as a therapy for migraine: "[I]n many of the skulls the holes show signs of healing and new growth of bone around the edges, indicating that the patients (victims?) survived the operation and lived for some years afterward" (Silverstein 4). Skulls historically tracing the practice have been found from prehistoric to modern sites in Sweden, Russia, the Pacific Islands, England (Forlag 1916), Kenya, Tanzania, southern Sudan, Somalia, Ethiopia (Margetts 1967), Alaska (Fortuine 1985), Greece (Arnott 1997), Peru, France, and Israel (Gross 1999). Each of these studies indicates trepanning as a treatment for migraine or headache. Graham Martin reports that as late as 1997, trepanning was still practiced for migraine among the Kinsii people in Kenya and Uganda:

> Probably a new source of pain in the scalp suppresses the old headache, by competing for, occupying and blocking, the same pain pathways to the brain, just as acupuncture or the old mustard plaster did. Probably most of the trepanned benefitted, because at least for a while, if the headache came back, some returned for a second or even third operation.
>
> (Martin 31)

This explains why some trepanned skulls have been discovered with so many holes that Forlag described them as "honeycombed" (150). The treatment was available to the young as well. F. P. Lisowski finds that "certainly children were trepanned" (667). Though, of course, this isn't depicted in fiction or film.

Within the rubric provided by the ubiquitous McGill pain questionnaire, migraine patients are likely to select adjectival forms of transitive verbs implicitly performed with weapons: piercing, pounding, shooting, boring, drilling, or stabbing. There is a salience to attacking the area of perceived pain even if it isn't a site of cause. Melanie Thernstrom reports meeting a man in Rwanda "with a pattern of burn marks encircling his forehead [who] had undergone a traditional treatment for migraines that had cured his chronic headaches" (299). When migraineurs feel their pain as if caused by a weapon but then imagine taking control of that weapon (as in holding the drill, ice pick) they insist on seeing their selves pitted against the body as a form of agency under the duress. A preservation of that self through self-violence, or through a willingness to intervene by ingesting drugs that promise to improve one's quality of life, even though they may have risks against later health and longevity, make better sense in this context.

Though seemingly self-destructive, such a position (of self-preservation through self-violence) necessitates an alternate notion of selfhood. Absolutist mind-body dualism of the Cartesian subject has been effectively dismantled by scholars like James Wilson, Cynthia Lewiecki-Wilson, Jack Richardson, and Jennifer Eisenhauer, who suggest that insisting upon a simplistic mind-body divide invites continued stigma and marginalization.[6] But the case of migraine can remind us why such reductive binarisms persist in the public imagination—they are discursively convenient ways of temporarily affirming a fortified sense of selfhood. And in the case of migraine, the physiological phenomenon in and of itself may preclude philosophizing, as indicated in the diagnostic narrative of one 12-year-old girl who distinguishes the severity and peculiar disconnection of migraine from other headaches because her head feels like "it has come off my body" (Stafstrom 2002).

The notion of an integrated embodied self has been questioned in cases of invisible, neurological, mental, and emotional impairment, and migraine offers a pertinent point in case that necessitates this nuance. This is partly because pain itself is, as Alyson Patsavas puts it, "often considered the most unincorporable disability experience" (206). Eleanor Kaufman uses (Nietszche's) migraine (via Pierre Klossowski) as her central example in the argument that "radical separation of mind and body" is necessary as a "defence" against certain illness experiences: "The execution of this powerful technique rests fundamentally on the disentangling of mind and body so that the mind can function as the strategizing spectator to the body's disempowerment" (136). In such a light the inner struggles of mind against body during migraine represent a method of subversive, "spectator" agency rather than a dismissal of bodymind integration or disability solidarity. Joanna Kempner writes, "Talking about the brain as a separate entity from oneself is a way of granting distance from one's disability," meaning the pain experience, not the political category, but

> [t]he separation between "I" and "my brain" is slippery and difficult to maintain. In the case of migraine, this separation requires that individuals sustain two different personalities – one that they use to define themselves and one that they use to describe their brains. I, for example, think of myself as an easygoing person, who happens to share a headspace with a difficult-to-manage brain.
>
> (100, 101)

Eula Biss describes a similar but impossible need to distinguish the self from the body during pain:

> I do not know how long I have been clenching my teeth when I notice that I am clinching my teeth. My mind, apparently, has not been with my body. I wonder why, when I most want to, I cannot seem to keep my mind from my body. I no longer know who I am, or if I am in charge of myself.
>
> (2007, 38)

By imagining the brain or body as separate from themselves, people in prolonged pain attempt to fortify the aspect of identity they can still imagine controlling.

Carla Cantor has written, "The rigid line between mental and physical is slowly dissolving, and someday the so-called Cartesian split will seem as ludicrous and arcane as the belief that the world is flat" (155). Yet, migraineurs persist in perceiving their minds and bodies at odds, though in changing terms. Justine Murison argues that the current "neuroscientific turn," which favors focusing on the body as the source for all mind experience, actually began as early as the 1840s in the United States, "providing both a vocabulary and a model for reconsidering the relation of the psyche and soma. It encourages scholars to consider the very *materiality* of the brain and nervous system as the location of complexity and creativity rather than the 'screen' of a deeper psyche" (29). Looking at nineteenth-century mesmerism as a "materialized spirituality," Murison has argued that public "cure" performances promised control of the body for those with "painful illnesses, from migraines and neuralgia to cancer" (30–31). Though such methods never became widely accepted, they represent early efforts to materialize migraine. For much of the twentieth century, however, migraine was seen by many as a somaticized disorder recurrent in particular personalities.

There has been a historic tendency of diagnosing "migraine personality" as nervous, creative, intelligent, and always sensitive. Of course this "sensitivity" is a symptom of organic origins now understood not as a personality issue, but the long tradition of blaming personality is deeply engrained. Hector Charles Cameron comprehensively secured this psychosomaticizing tendency in his 1922 edition of *The Nervous Child*. Bernard Myers continued in this tradition of pro-filing, writing in 1925 that "headache, and migraine, may be all due to vasomo-tor disturbance. Hypersensitiveness of taste, hearing, sight, smell, and touch are usually present. . . . No wonder that as babies they are difficult to feed" (158). In 1955 Russell DeJong argued definitively that

> the attacks are in most instances precipitated by psychological factors. The patient who is subject to migraine has certain personality characteristics. The attacks . . . are more frequent in the "thinkers" that is, in the professional and semi-professional groups, than in the doers."
>
> (56)

Somewhat sympathetically, Cedric Harvey et al. wrote in 1956 that in diagnosing migraine early,

> [w]e shall save children from mistaken appendix operations . . . cut down the number of pairs of spectacles and tonsillectomies suggested for school-children. We shall spare many children the humiliation of being regarded by teachers as physical ne'er-do-wells because of their mysterious periodic prostrating bouts.
>
> (1430)

In 1975 the *British Medical Journal* included an unattributed editorial on cyclical vomiting (an early indication of migraine), which stated that "the children with recurrent abdominal pains tend as a group to be more timid, anxious, tense, and fussy than those who are symptom free; they also tend to be over-conscientious and to be bad mixers" (anon 459). And in 1993 K. R. Merikangas et al. would still argue that "migraineurs had greater levels of neuroticism than did those without migraine, but no difference emerged for extraversion or psychoticism" (188). In fact, the only certainty in such emphases is that migraine is proven to be comorbid with anxiety and depression, which of course, could just as likely result from severe episodic pain. Studies indicate clear environmental factors that essentializations of "migraine personality" are designed to ignore.

By the 1990s neuroscientists dubbed an emerging era[7] of inquiry and advance "the Age of the Brain." Neurologists and neuroscientists isolated the causes of migraine in cortical hyperexcitability and central sensitization (Dodick 2006), even capturing the process through neuroimaging (Woods et al. 1994, Iacoboni 2009). Joanna Kempner documents that in turn people with migraine reconfigured their disease biodeterministically in order to legitimate the disorder as a "brain disease," which, rather than being totally affirmative, simply resulted in a semantic restructuring of the same legitimacy crisis: "shifting the blame from 'character' to the 'brain' does not remove migraine from a person's identity" (73). As a compensatory narrative, for the delegitimized person with an invisible impairment, being able to say one has a "brain disease" rather than a psychosomatic personality problem has a sympathetic appeal, but it fails to address holistic experience by focusing solely on the body, unfortunately reaffirming profit-driven efforts to treat migraine through trial-and-error "off-label" prescribing of anticonvulsants prophylactically. Many of these drugs can have dire side effects and offer less relief than abortive meds.

Even conceptualizing migraine as a brain disease leaves too much room for medicated persons to be socially blamed rather than helped, especially in light of concerns surrounding the boom in psychotherapeutic and anticonvulsant pharmacology. When antimedication psychiatrist Peter Breggin visited the campus where I work for a guest lecture, he opened with and often repeated the mantra, "Drugs kill the brain," advocating empathetic counseling instead. Ironically, he was being far from empathetic to the many persons in the audience who were either medicated or medicating others for conditions that may be overprescribed but have few treatment options. Like many he seemed to be unaware that taking drugs is often the last resort for patients who have tried countless, failed coping methods (or don't have access to the same counseling services that Breggin's wealthy clientele do) and have decided that their symptoms are worse than drug side effects and long-term risks.

In contrast to Breggin's reductionist dismissal, Margaret Price provides an embodied rhetorical analysis of mental disability, explaining the relationship between prescriber and patient in this more empowering way: "I consider myself the agent and director of my treatments; for example, I interviewed and discarded psychiatrists until I found one who agrees with my approach to my bodymind" (11). When others, like Breggin, think with no more nuance than "drugs kill the brain," they are overlooking the fact that this is one of the risks many patients feel they have no choice but to take. We should be developing more and better choices, rather than taking away the few (albeit flawed) choices available for empowering persons with mental impairments and chronic disease. Those who disparage all medicalized identity overlook this reality of invisible disability. The perspective of persons with mental impairment surveyed by Margaret Price echoes a practical counterbalance to the blaming of impaired and medicated individuals: "Despite their awareness of the problems posed by diagnosis, all of the participants expressed an attendant awareness of its importance in their material lives—in particular, its relevance to the medications and quality of care they can access" (215). Diagnosis and treatment are a part of the everyday, material lives of many persons living with chronic or fluctuating impairments. Understanding them is a necessary investment toward understanding those who know the stakes intimately.

It is also possible to imagine one's self and pain as separate without oversimplifying the (dis)connection between mind and body. We can learn, for example, from persons with prosthesis and transplant experiences, that, as Margrit Shildrick has argued, "the body is *always* a stranger to itself," because "all bodies swarm with and are—in the normal course of events—sustained in health by, a multitude of putatively alien others" (275, 278). If we look at our bodies on the level of microorganisms, as comprised by an inestimable and constantly changing multitude of microbes (like digestive bacteria), we can see that the fictive disembodiment demanded of the person in pain is just another way of imagining our "selves" as episodic hosts to neuro-determined ruptures in our experience. If we see our bodies as multiply constituted, and the mind as a part and consequence of that constitution, the usefulness of Price's preferred term, "bodymind," is more apparent. Our experience is always on a continuum. The self was never situated in just mind or body.

Neuroresearcher Antonio Damasio points out that even in the "age of the brain" we can imagine a unified self that transcends the sorting of body or mind:

> The appearance of a gulf between mental states and physical/biological phenomena comes from the large disparity between two bodies of knowledge – the good understanding of mind we have achieved through centuries of introspection and the efforts of cognitive science versus the incomplete neural specification we have achieved through the efforts of neuroscience. But there is no reason to expect that neurobiology cannot bridge the gulf. Nothing indicates that we have reached an edge of the abyss that would separate, in principle, the mental from the neural.
>
> (115)

Of course, for Damasio the unifying mode of inquiry is scientific. And there's another bias in his approach. The hyperspecialization of neurosciences and neurology often leaves migraine in a liminal position in spite of how commonly it is experienced. Michael D. Gershon, who scientifically legitimized what Ayurvedic practitioners have known for thousands of years, has popularized understanding of the autonomic functions of the gut (enteric nervous system) as a "second brain," which has important implications for our concepts of migraine and selfhood. Gershon points out that "[n]euroscientists, whose horizon ends at the holes in the skull, are continually amazed to find that the structure and component cells of the enteric nervous system are more akin to those of the brain than to those of any other peripheral organ" (xiii). Neurologists, likewise, seldom look below the neck when treating patients for migraine, which is a serious short-sidedness when it comes to a disorder that, contrary to popular belief, is a whole-body experience with pronounced abdominal symptoms. Giulia Enders has made the implications of this finding even more accessible to a general audience in her book *Gut: The Inside Story of Our Most Underrated Organ* (2015). Not only does the existence of a "second brain" indicate the need for greater attention to the role of the gut in migraine research, but Enders suggests that the Age of the Brain may well give way to an Age of the Second Brain, changing the way we define our sense of self: "Our self is created in our head and our gut—no longer just in language but increasingly also in the lab" (125). When one considers a migraine patient intersecting with science by communicating with a medical practitioner, we find something even more phenomenologically complicated. I'll look more closely at these repercussions in the next chapter, but for now suffice it to say that wherever the "self" is rooted, during an attack, a migraineur is still likely to cast the conflict as one between the self and the body (whether focused on the brain, the gut, or both) no matter how aware one is that one's self would not exist without the brain.

Determinism pervades literary descriptions of migraine, often conveying the sense of migraine as intractable foe. Joan Didion, who was eight when she first experienced migraine, writes that "[o]nce an attack is under way, however, no drug touches it" (169–170). Though many have depended upon opiates, they are ultimately ineffective in aborting a migraine attack, in which the pain will escalate until one sleeps. In her "Migraine Sonnets," Marilyn Hacker describes the attack as inevitable, intractable: "The night progresses like chronic disease, symptom by symptom, sentences without pardon" (188). Successful abortive medication, especially the "triptan revolution" in the 1990s, would change this for some and reaffirm for many that migraine is a disorder of the brain, one that we can control to some extent. Patrick Humphrey writes that

> the discovery of sumatriptan confirmed, once and for all, that migraine truly is an organic disease and not just the figment of imagination of "neurotic" patients. Indeed, in the early days of sumatriptan's availability, it was hailed as a diagnostic for whether or not a patient's headache was migrainous in origin.
> (685)

Some cling to this biodeterministic model too tightly, at the expense of ignoring pain behavior, addiction, or alternate therapies that can aid in the success of aborting attacks and in some cases reduce their frequency.

For the most part, the intricacies of perception and bodily maintenance are detectable only between the lines of literary depictions. As Virginia Woolf has noted, literature is preoccupied with the screen of the mind. Most literary representations of migraine are not as violent and body conscious as *That Beautiful Somewhere*, but they do incorporate clues as to the embodied realities of migraineurs and material methods for coping of their times. And in their incorporation of social and biological beliefs about migraine, they transmit stereotypes or can legitimize the migraining bodymind.

Diagnostic criticism and medical literature

One of the most popular legitimizing techniques found in medical and popular writing about migraine is to list and laud famous migraineurs whose personal authority legitimizes migraine by association—from Ulysses S. Grant and Karl Marx to Elvis Presley[8]—in an effort to show just how common the disorder is, but also with a compensatory nod to the migraineur-reader, to show that he or she is in good company. One of the most famous of these, and certainly the most cited literary migraineur, is Charles Dodgson, penname Lewis Carroll (a bibliography of works on migraine that include references to Carroll and often even John Tenniel's illustrations would fill a very lengthy book). Literary criticism, medical literature, and popular appropriations have created an author function to support a biodeterministic mythology of migraine around Carroll. Some suggest that the vanishing Cheshire Cat, Alice's shrinking and growing, and tricky time perceptions reflect the author's experience with aura (Lippmann 1952, Rolak 1991, van Vugt 1994, Bral 1999, Larner 2004, Restak 2006). Others, like Selwyn Goodacre, contest the intentional fallacy (though not in those terms) and object to the extent that Carroll's imagination is slighted by the suggestion that his literary inspiration was thoroughly neurological:

> Lewis Carroll certainly suffered from migraine. Commentators have seized on this with delight. . . . Unfortunately for this attractive idea, the first record of an attack is in 1885 (20 years after "Alice") when Carroll says quite definitely that this was only the second time.
>
> (236)

Lewis Carroll's primary experience with migraine was probably with aura, not pain (Murray), so these legitimacy narratives tend to romanticize aura. There is strong evidence that he experienced aura, proven by a famous drawing in which negative scotoma is clearly present. Later in life this was accompanied by headache, and in a diary entry written during his fifties he admits that an eye-problem may have been "bilious-headache" all along, just without the pain (Podoll and Robinson 1999, 1366). But critics go to absurd lengths in order to insist a direct causal relationship between Carroll's own migraine experience and the multiple auratic features of his fiction. Richard Restak quotes Norwegian neurologist Jill Gordon Klee asserting rightfully that most likely Carroll had experienced aura earlier in life without headache, but dubiously speculating that "he did not dare record these manifestations," which to anyone familiar with Carroll's published and unpublished writing, is clearly projecting motivations that don't fit (quoted in Restak 308). Most migraineurs, though sometimes frightened the first time they experience aura, in fact usually become familiar quickly with their altered perception, especially when the alterations are identical in subsequent attacks. When Restak agrees with Klee, "Perhaps he, too, feared being thought insane," he is protesting just enough to reveal his own over-investment in diagnostically materializing Carroll's literary creations as neurological symptoms (308). It is now known that diverse perceptual distortions and hallucinations are associated with a range of neurological differences and imbalances caused by acute or chronic experience with illness (or, to be discussed below, drug use).

An aura in which proportions (micropsia and macropsia) and depth perception are distorted is even named Alice in Wonderland syndrome. Once thought to be infrequent in children (Golden 517), it is now thought that the syndrome, "like migraine, appears to be more common in young people, even children" and, as with Dodgson, often occurs independent of headache, with epilepsy or encephalitis (Rolak 649). One migraineur I interviewed, Jessica Benzel, whose attacks began around age nine, described among her other prodromal symptoms, like speech problems, numbness, and temporary paralysis, her experience with Alice in Wonderland syndrome:

> I feel like I'm in a fish bowl. Sometimes it feels like my arms are way too long, and sometimes my voice sounds like my ears are plugged (I can especially hear it when I say the "S" sound). If I'm not sure whether or not I'm getting a migraine, I hold out my hand to judge how long I think my arm looks.
>
> (personal interview)

Certainly such phenomena resemble Alice's perceptions (see figure 3.1).

For children experiencing aura for the first time, Andrew Levy recommends reading Lewis Carroll:

> There may be no better literary representation of migraine in history – not the pain but the distorted and escalating sensibility. It is the first book a migraineur needs to read to dissolve the alienation; it is the first book someone without migraines needs to read if he or she is curious about what it's like. And it is the first book to use as evidence if one wants to argue that migraine taps a worldview, a deep pattern, available to migraineur and nonmigraineur alike.
>
> (106–107)

Perhaps it's no coincidence that the first serious book I bought as a child with my own money was a paperback copy of Martin Gardner's *Annotated Alice*. Of course the *Alice* books[9] don't provide bibliotherapy for migraine pain, but for that today's child migraineur can turn to *Harry Potter* for a hint of affirmation in its headache-ridden hero.

At the intersection of medical narratives and literary criticism is a fascinating tradition of diagnostic reductionism attempting to legitimate migraine but sometimes backfiring with transparent romanticization. Siri Hustvedt reports that William James used the term "medical materialism" for the "tendency to reduce artistic, religious, or philosophic achievements to bodily ailment" (2012, 29). What really interests me in the case of Lewis Carroll and migraines is the extent to which reading his work as migraine literature is taken up in popular writing in this reductive manner, to the extent that the *Alice* books, multiple websites will tell you, were "inspired by" migraine and aura. Andrew Levy puts such oversimplifications

quite dull and stupid for things to go on in the common way.

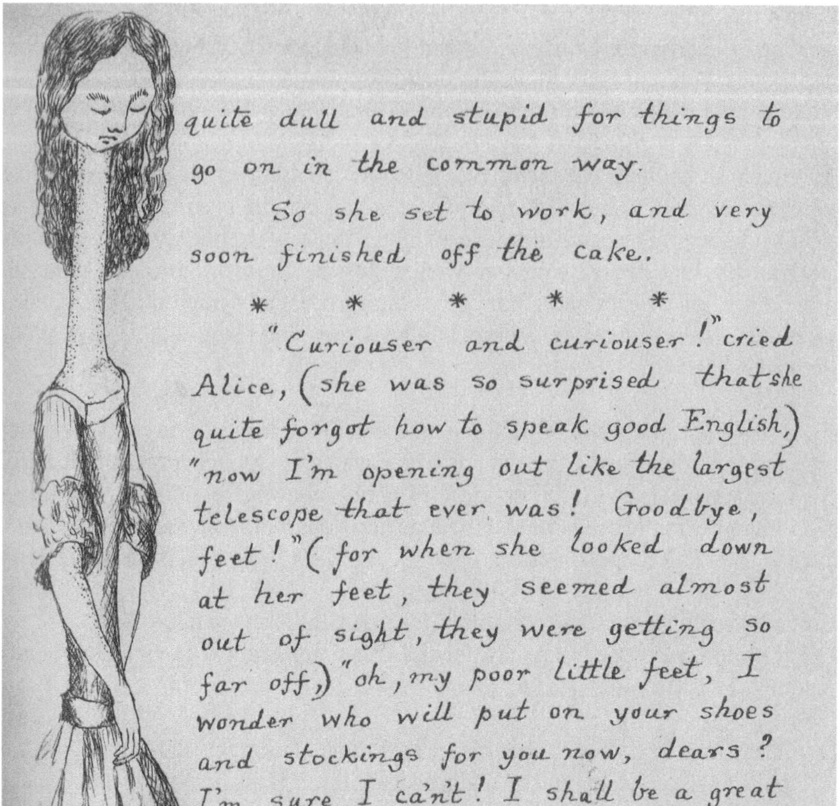

So she set to work, and very soon finished off the cake.

*   *   *   *   *

"Curiouser and curiouser!" cried Alice, (she was so surprised that she quite forgot how to speak good English,) "now I'm opening out like the largest telescope that ever was! Goodbye, feet!" (for when she looked down at her feet, they seemed almost out of sight, they were getting so far off,) "oh, my poor little feet, I wonder who will put on your shoes and stockings for you now, dears? I'm sure I can't! I shall be a great deal too far off to bother myself about you: you must manage the best way you can— but I must be kind to them", thought Alice, "or perhaps they won't walk the way I want to go! Let me see: I'll give them a new pair of boots every Christmas."

And she went on planning to herself how she would manage it:

Figure 3.1 Lewis Carroll, *Alice's Adventures Underground* © The British Library Board, Add. 46700, f.7

aptly to rest: "There have been tens of millions, even hundreds of millions, with migraine: there has been only one *Alice in Wonderland*" (101). Yet, as Justine Murison suggests, the materializing lean observable in earlier attitudes toward migraine existed in the nineteenth century, and it clearly didn't stop then. The meeting of body and mind in brain science is a perfect example—popular interpretations simplify with a biodeterministic spin. Neuroscientist Antonio Damasio put this succinctly when interviewed by Lone Frank:

> Journalists simplify the research until it becomes unrecognizable and make everything into a story about here's the brain center for this and the brain center for that. They want to sell an easy message that these "centers" control and define us. The idea is easy to communicate, and it is easy for the public to swallow it.
>
> (quoted in Frank 171)

Youth are particularly ill served by such reductionism, as in the ubiquitous generalization that just because the frontal lobes are still developing, children are not developed enough to make reliable decisions—never mind that even neuroscientists don't know enough about the frontal lobes for such absolutism and will be the first to tell you so.

Neuroscience has played an important role in legitimating migraine, as in the neuroimaging that proved one could witness the decrease in cerebral blood flow in process if caught during aura (Woods et al. 1994, Iacobani 2009). But visual proofs are often lacking in nuance. In *Picturing Personhood*, Joseph Dumit argues this in the case of the "persuasiveness of visual images" in the courtroom during expert testimonies: "The paradox of expert images in a trial is that if they are legible, then they should not need interpretation, but if they need interpretation, then they should probably not be shown to juries" (112). As the progress of queer and disability politics has shown, visibility is a powerful tool, but what is perceivable still requires explanation—seeing doesn't mean knowing.

Literary criticism, an interpretive endeavor, is such a process. And when a seemingly subjective practice is bolstered with the clout of science the result can be seductively convincing, reducing all creative or nonrealistic elements of culture to a biologically knowable cause—rooting flights of fancy in the body through medicalizing explanations. Take, for example, the fact that Lewis Carroll was interested in the occult and claimed to believe in fairies (Cohen 369). By the logic of determinism, this too could be connected to his migraine experience. Folklorist R. U. Sayce argued in 1934 that belief in fairies can be "shaped" by hallucination caused by eye problems like cataract, brain injury, "Various illnesses such as epilepsy and migraine," or drugs (105). With just a dangerous amount of knowledge, reductionism abounds in responses to literature like Carroll's. As Kenneth Kidd puts it, "[S]ource texts do not always authorize their aftertexts" (73). My favorite example, and a pertinent one to Carroll's posthumously pseudo-medicalized identity, is Thomas Fensch's *Alice in Acidland* (1970). Fensch argues, in the introduction to his wackily annotated version of the original, that "[c]ritics who would claim that Lewis Carroll originally had no idea of hallucinogenic chemicals may be mistaken in their interpretation of his personality. . . . He may have been, in fact, the original proponent of the use of these drugs" (1970, 12–13). Lewis Carroll has been a popular figure in psychedelic culture—an association emphasized particularly by John Lennon,[10] who insisted that Carroll be included on the cover of *Sgt. Pepper's Lonely Hearts Club Band* (1967). Fensch admits, "It is doubtful that [Carroll] ever knew of the nineteenth-century equivalent of LSD, but *Alice in Wonderland* echoes the confused, surrealistic world—the world of the LSD trip" (1968, 424). From the standpoint of literary scholarship, this would be considered the worst kind of self-indulgent anachronism and intentional fallacy, and of course even Fensch knows that his foundational premise is completely untenable (he does not mention what the nineteenth-century "equivalent of LSD" would be). But he is making a link between Carroll, hallucination, and drugs that has some relevance[11] to the material history of migraine.

A precursor to today's triptans, LSD belongs to a class of substances that are "the most potent anti-serotonin substances known," and its derivative, methysergide "has been used prophylactically by a number of workers in the treatment of migraine" (Elithorn 412). In fact, when Albert Hofmann first produced LSD in 1938,[12] he was working with ergot to create a "serotonin antagonist without psychedelic effects" for aborting migraine attacks (Grof 22). Ergot, a hallucinogenic and often dangerous[13] fungus that grows on rye, now considered responsible for the Salem witch trials and many earlier cases of European witch hunts, has been used medically since the early nineteenth century to induce labor and stop bleeding after childbirth (Tansey 195). But ergot was most certainly known to have therapeutic value much earlier, as evidenced in a Nordic poem from the eighth or ninth century (Stein 392–393). Ragnar Stein writes,

> [T]he constrictor effect on blood vessels, so intensively used in our century against migraine, was known to Nordic medieval doctors. The prescription probably began in the 9th or 10th century and is the first medical use of ergot alkaloids that I have come across.
>
> (393)

A truly interdisciplinary discovery.

More germane to the historic context in which Lewis Carroll was writing, ergot was first recommended for the treatment of migraine in 1868,[14] three years after the publication of *Alice's Adventures in Wonderland* and three years before *Through the Looking-Glass* (Tfelt-Hansen 753). Of course, I'm not suggesting that Carroll took ergot or was even aware of it, but instead want to stress that hallucination is hardly unique to migraine or any one particular substance. Cocaine, which Sigmund Freud took for his migraine, has been found to produce "herringbone" and "zig-zag" hallucinations similar to scintillating and fortification migraine aura. Ronald Siegel "hypothesizes that cocaine, migraines, hallucinogens, photostimulation and electrical current all produce the same type of 'excitation' of the central nervous system" (quoted in Greenberg 190–191). Carroll and his critics would have a range of experiences to interpret along seemingly shared idiosyncratic lines.

In *Touching a Nerve: The Self as Brain*, Patricia Churchland recalls the experience of one of her friends in high school,

> who suffered a weeklong catastrophic migraine every spring. In the days just prior to the onset of the migraine, she said that at night she usually had the experience of feeling that she was very, *very* tiny – about the size of a hornet – in a massively huge bed. The sensation did not alarm her because she knew it was a "brain thing" that would disappear. And it did. What did bother her was that her miniaturization experience reliably augured the migraine to come.
>
> (75)

The fact that such experience, Alice in Wonderland syndrome, and its inverse, Lilliputian hallucination, both have literary names speaks to how poetically they generate fascination. But this testimony reminds us that the pain to come, not the aura itself, produces dread of the next attack. There is *nothing* poetic about the pain.

Fictional migraine

Migraine aura, particularly visual hallucinations, have attracted much artistic, popular, and medical attention. There is something mythical about aura, as Siri Hustvedt points out: "The content of hallucinations must surely be at once personal and cultural," indicated by the prevalence of folkloric visualizations like her own of Paul Bunyan and others she's heard of, like Martians and cartoon characters (34). Yet aura are not only a brief part of migraine episodes (lasting 5 to 30 minutes in the prodromal phase), but most migraineurs don't even experience aura. Migraine with aura, which affects "one in four" migraineurs, "is characterized by a relatively short duration (under twelve hours) compared with the common migraine headache (up to four days)" (Beil 27, WHO 326). With all those extra hours of pain, poor "common" migraine apparently doesn't get any more interesting. "Classical migraine," now called migraine with aura, steals the show—with aura taking the spotlight.

With a similarly disproportionate focus, the tradition of literary representations of migraine is full of symbolic erasures of pain. Pain is explained away as unworthy of much concern. The literary migraineur is usually a flawed character, whose "migraine personality" makes her or him just unsympathetic enough to blame for the pain. The literary *child* migraineur exists, if at all, to reflect the pain or flaws of another. Too often, pain itself becomes simply a metaphor.

Perhaps the most original use of migraine in literature occurs when migraineur Mikhail Bulgakov (see Zayas et al.) makes migraine an important deciding factor in some of the most sensational scenes from religious history by foregrounding the olfactory aura (smelling of rose oil) and migraine pain he attributes to Pontius Pilate as he interrogates the prisoner Yeshua (Jesus) in *The Master and Margarita* (written from 1928 to 1940 but not fully published until 1973). Pilate feels the pain coming on and repeatedly thinks of suicide: "Suddenly the thought of poison flashed seductively through the procurator's aching head. . . . Poison, give me poison." (17). He is aware that he could speed through this interview to judgment in order to seek relief sooner:

> [A]s an agonizing wave of nausea swept over him, the procurator realized that the simplest way to get this strange miscreant off his balcony was with two words, "Hang him." Get rid of the escort too, leave the colonnade, go inside the palace, order the room darkened, collapse on the bed, ask for some cold water, call piteously for the dog Banga, and complain to him about his hemicrania.
>
> (17)

But as he speaks to the wise prisoner he senses that Yeshua could heal him, again tipping the scales of justice based on his pain. Yeshua tells Pilate,

> The truth is, first of all, that your head aches, so badly, in fact, that you're having fainthearted thoughts about death . . . That I, at this moment, am your unwilling executioner upsets me. You can't think about anything and the only thing you want is to call your dog, the only creature, it seems, to whom you are attached. But your sufferings will soon end, and your headache will pass.
>
> (17)

Pilate asks Yeshua, "Tell the truth, are you a great physician?" (18). Though he is not, Yeshua consoles Pilate that the weather will change shortly, and his pain will lessen. And so Pilate's and Yeshua's fates are sealed.

Migraine is realistically recurrent in *Fortunata and Jacinta: Two Stories of Married Women* (1886–1887), by Benito Pérez Galdós, also a migraineur. His characters, Maximiliano Rubín and his brothers, all have migraines, but Maxi's get the most focus, perhaps most amusingly the attack he gets on his wedding night.[15] He tries to conceal his illness until it is apparent to the wedding party, who discuss his condition: "Everyone looked piteously at the poor migraine victim and some of the guests suggested extravagant remedies" (392). Maxi's gluttonous brother, Nicolás, chimes in:

> It's a family illness. . . . Nothing helps. I've had such bad ones that the days I had them I couldn't help but compare myself to Saint Peter when he had the axe in his head. For some time now I've been curing them with ham.
>
> (392)

Galdós incorporates diagnostic detail, like Maxi's vomiting, "epileptic tingling," and his distinctive progression of pain from the right side to left, which give an appreciated measure of idiosyncratic credibility (393). The prescription is especially measured:

> [D]on't forget the flask of laudanum.[16] Fortunata, go get it. When I go to bed, I'll try to sleep, and if I can't, put six drops – measure carefully, now – six drops of this medicine in a glass of water and give it to me to drink.
>
> (393)

Is it wish-fulfillment that inspired Galdós to make Maxi a pharmacist?

Naturalistic detail aside, the novel includes features that, from today's perspective, are the bane of migraine literature: the term for migraine Galdós uses, "jaqueca," is used liberally throughout the book just as "migraine" is freely misapplied in English—referring to a problem, a conflict, or even nagging—as in "that blasted Fortunata, who had given her so many headaches" (456). More relevant to the argument of this book, however, is that the brothers' migraine is depicted as

> physiologically emblematic of the ongoing dysfunction of the home where they grew up. Though they may manifest themselves in different aspects, their headaches witness that the sins of the fathers, or more particularly of the mother, are literally visited on the heads of the children.
>
> (Larsen 413)

Unfortunately, the critic who makes this observation, Kevin Larsen, seems to be including the mother's "promiscuity" as a possible cause of dysfunction (the brothers each have a different father). Another critic, Angel Garma, blames Maxi's premature birth and his mother's inability to breast-feed (cited in Larsen, 413). Such mother-blaming draws us closer to the more common stereotypes of literary migraine so familiar in the form of those ubiquitous nineteenth-century hysterics and malingerers, and Galdós is not immune to this prejudice.

Though Maxi's migraines are presented as real, completely legitimate, deserving of sympathy and careful treatment, his wife simply fakes one:

> [A]fter lunch and when Maxi had left for the pharmacy, Fortunata was so afraid of an angry outburst that she faked a migraine. Tying a cloth around her head, she shut herself up in her room and went to bed. . . . [H]er thoughts blurred in grief and pain and finally drowsiness overtook her.
>
> (609)

Here Galdós taps into and perpetuates the easy flow of nineteenth-century female stereotypes—women's complaints can't be trusted, "pain" is some kind of vague malaise, and because they are invisible, migraines are easy to fake thus might not always be real.

John Steinbeck, who had a medically precarious childhood,[17] made the invisibility and resulting socially perceived ambiguity of migraine one of the main themes of *The Wayward Bus* (1947). Like most literary migraineurs, Steinbeck's example is a woman and mother, Bernice, usually called merely Mrs. Pritchard. On one hand, her migraines are described in terms that suggest they are genuine, inevitable, and uncontrollable:

> [H]er headaches . . . were dreadful. They twisted her face and reduced her to a panting, sweating, grinning, quivering blob of pain. . . . [Her husband] could feel it all over his body, and the doctor said there was nothing to do about it. They injected calcium and they gave her sedatives. The headaches usually

came when she was nervous and when things, through no fault of her own, were not going well.

(175–176)

But one can see early on that the perspective is tilted toward how her husband feels about her attacks rather than sympathetically focused on her. And though what is stated is that Bernice "was very brave. She tried to muffle her screams with a pillow," what we are shown and made to feel is quite unsympathetic (176). Through her husband's viewpoint we see her migraine legitimated as very real and debilitating, yet the dominant viewpoint of the novel is to see him as both overly concerned with her care, henpecked and emasculated by the burden, and sex-starved by her apparently migraine-related frigidity. One contemporary reviewer, Harrison Smith, pegged it perfectly and in such a hostile manner that it leaves no doubt as to the novel's effect: "Mr. Pritchard is dirty-minded, boastful, dishonest, and hag-ridden by his wife; she has remained an aging little girl who has doubtless by immaculate conception produced a child, and who brings her family to heel by imaginary illnesses" (quoted in McElrath et al., 294). Indeed Mr. Pritchard infantilizes his wife, whom he calls "little girl" and smothers with attention to her potential pains (190, 228). In fact, he views her as an embodiment of the nineteenth-century stereotyped hysteric, which in a perverse way reaffirms her femininity and class to him: "Mr. Pritchard considered his wife's shortcomings as a woman the attributes of a lady" (53). Like the fainting ladies of old (think, for example, of the women in *Dracula*), Bernice Pritchard is attributed with a helpless sexual invitation complicated by being desexed: "Mr. Pritchard didn't bother her much in bed—very seldom, in fact. But in a curious way he tied up his occasional lust and his loss of self-control with her headaches" (176). Mrs. Pritchard is something of a non-character who merely reflects her husband's man pain and the psychological dysfunctions of her family, a barely fleshed-out version of the cliché excuse, "not tonight, honey." Even so, it still comes as quite a shock (and sorry for the spoiler if all this actually makes you want to read the book), when, spurred on by the comments of others who make him see his uxoriousness as emasculating (237, 239), Mr. Pritchard rapes her. When she complains that he is tearing her dress he justifies his action and blames her for the necessary violence of his attack: "'I bought it, didn't I? I'm tired of being treated like a sick cat'" (240). But he is only *sick* in a figurative or moral sense of the word—it is his wife's illness that is *not* imaginary.

In spite of Steinbeck's legitimizing details (like Galdós, he uses a naturalist's eye) about Bernice's migraine, such as prodromal experience, like the "telegraph poles whipping by as little blows on her eyes" (120), the novel ultimately leaves the reader with a shockingly unsympathetic view, and the plot eventually delegitimizes migraine pain (or uses its presumably accepted status as an "imaginary illness" to delegitimize her) by focusing strictly on how the attacks negatively affect those around her: "They filled a room and a house. They got into everyone around her. Mr. Pritchard could feel one of her headaches through walls" (175). Rather than situating us in the mind of Mrs. Pritchard, Steinbeck leaves her completely undeveloped psychologically, instead knowable only as a reflection of her family's psychology.

This influence is reflected most through the stereotyped migraineur's inability to nurture when ill. She is the textbook example of the culturally imposed guilt placed on migraining mothers. Mildred, Bernice's daughter, views her mother's attacks as "too opportunely" timed, a "curse," and "pure sham" (207, 177). But the biggest sham in the book is the subtly self-negating sympathy offered in descriptions like this one: "They seemed to be selfish, these headaches, and yet they were not. The pain was real. No one could simulate such agonizing pain" (176). Ultimately Bernice is to blame for her actual pain and the metaphorical pain of her family. Her daughter expresses the view that comes to dominate the book (and is even worse in the 1957 film adaptation[18]): "You're going to get a headache and punish us. One of your fake headaches" (207). The perverse idea that pain is selfish speaks to the extent to which migraining mothers are seen as transgressing their obligatory role of nurturer, but it also reveals the subtler cultural refusal to recognize that pain is not fully within the migraineur's control.

These accusatory cultural stereotypes have had lasting detrimental consequences for women with migraine. The migraineur mentioned previously who committed suicide when her heroin shots became regulated and denied was heartlessly dismissed as a nervous case: "Such mishaps were dismissed as exceptional and to be expected with any drug in highly strung individuals" (Dormandy 197). Stephen Kandall writes, in *Substance and Shadow: Women and Addiction in the United States*, of how blaming drug-using mothers, in particular, has had a lasting effect. The flip side, ironically, is the mother-guilt used to sell "mother's little helpers" of all generations. Joanna Kempner details the many ways in which antimigraine pharmaceuticals are still advertised by not only stereotyping migraine as a woman's 'complaint' but tapping and aggravating mother-guilt as a predominant sales technique:

> The latent message, on the one hand, confirms that migraine is a women's disorder that disrupts feminine efforts to care for others. . . . The pill does more than treat her migraine symptoms; it transforms her into a more reasonable, dependable person.
>
> (126)

In such narratives, the migraining mother is damned either way—a selfish addict or failure at what matters most.

Ian McEwan's *Atonement* (2001) offers a kinder representation of the migraining mother through sheer descriptive power and by focusing on the attack from the migraineur's perspective, not simply her family's, but it also leaves the primary bias unquestioned. Closely following the slow and painful progress of an attack in the novel's matriarch, Emily Tallis, McEwan effectively portrays the banality of sitting out, suffering, and waiting for the attack to run its course, beginning with her aura:

> She was not in pain, not yet, but she was retreating before its threat. There were illuminated points in her vision, little pinpricks, as though the worn

fabric of the visible world was being held up against a far brighter light. She felt in the top right corner of her brain a heaviness, the inert body weight of some curled and sleeping animal.

(60)

Less represented features, like phonophobia and photophobia, are concretely brought to the reader's awareness: "What to others would have been a muffling was to her alert senses, which were fine-tuned like the cat's whiskers of an old wireless, an almost unbearable amplification" (63). Like Maxi and Mrs. Pritchard, Emily strategizes for coping, planning to avoid "exposure to unadulterated sunlight" as "even the diminishing rays of early evening could provoke an attack. The sunglasses would have to be found" (67). In multiple examples, the pain is described in terms of an imagined weapon: "She lay rigidly apprehensive, held at knifepoint, knowing that fear would not let her sleep and that her only hope was in keeping still" (61), "knifing pains would obliterate all thought" (60), and more revealing of her class and consumerism,

> the fear of pain kept her in place. At worst, unrestrained, a matching set of sharpened kitchen knives would be drawn across her optic nerve, and then again, with a greater downward pressure, and she would be entirely shut in and alone. Even groaning increased the agony.
>
> (63)

In his attention to detail, McEwan meets clinical precision with poetic power, but he also evokes the ladylike image of migraine as a luxury only those with wealth and housewifely duties can afford. As Joanna Kempner has argued, the archetype of the migraineur as an affluent housewife suggests the disorder is "temporary and distinctly bourgeois" (116, 131). Not only does this reaffirm inaccurate sexist and classist[19] stereotypes associated with migraine, but it couches the subtler assumption that it is not truly debilitating.

In *Atonement*, McEwan adds a decidedly more concrete and original spin to his retreading of migraine stereotypes in his extended metaphor comparing an attack to "some curled sleeping animal," "the black-furred creature," and "her animal tormentor" (60, 62, 66). Rather than assigning her migraine attack sentient intentionality, "It bore her no malice, this animal, it was indifferent to her misery" (60). This conceit reminds the reader of her connectedness to nonhuman animals through her vulnerability (a theme I'll investigate further in my final chapters). But the more dominant theme of the chapter devoted to Emily's attack is the toll it takes on her ability to nurture. Like Steinbeck, McEwan (inadvertently?) slips in the reflection of migraine on Emily as a failed mother whose disorder distracts her from her nurturing obligation: "Illness had stopped her giving her children all a mother should" (62–63). Or perhaps this is the character's focalized thought and the author sympathetically views her migraine as an expression of the strain from these duties, though she is nonetheless defined according to them:

Habitual fretting about her children, her husband, her sister, the help, had rubbed her senses raw; migraine, mother love and, over the years, many hours of lying still on her bed, had distilled from this sensitivity a sixth sense, a tentacular awareness that reached out from the dimness and moved through the house, unseen and all-knowing.

(63)

Certainly these literary migraining mothers are consistent with the extent to which migraine has been feminized, and so delegitimized along gendered lines. But they also speak to the ways in which our cultural stereotypes and literary figurations eclipse children who are also affected by the disorder.

The focus on mothers shifts attention entirely from their children, who, by the logic of medical knowledge (if we treat the fictional characters as realistic yet hypothetical persons) have a higher chance of inheriting the disorder and an increased likelihood of experiencing attacks in childhood. One migraining mother (and mother of a migraineur) I interviewed, Carrie Crockett, noted McEwan's oversight:

[T]he mother in Ian McEwan's *Atonement* suffers from terrible migraines that he describes wonderfully. When I read the chapter for the first time, however, one of the thoughts that crossed my mind is how lucky this woman was to have the ability to sit, alone, in a darkened room, until the pain had passed. Our kids – kids like Annecy [her daughter] – do not have this type of luxury.

(email)

While, as a migraining mother and reader, Carrie appreciated McEwan's depiction, as the mother of a child migraineur, she noticed one of the damaging effects of such stereotyping—it makes it easier to ignore exceptions to the fictional rule. Joanna Kempner warns that such characterizations establish "the commonsense notion that migraine is a condition that affects a particular kind of person—a white, middle-class woman—a construction that simultaneously stigmatizes the person with migraine, while rendering invisible other people with migraine" (109). Indeed, working-class and nonwhite migraineurs are invisible in fiction, an oversight redressed in my next chapter. But the gendering of migraine persists even in medical accounts. When we essentialize impairments as experienced by women, we are not just rigidly gendering them; we also make it more difficult to recognize the early impact on many of those affected, women and men, when they first need help—as children. Though migraine is a legacy illness experienced by many throughout the life span (as suggested in figure 3.2), migraine in children is all but ignored in fiction.

This oversight occurs even in children's books, where one might expect more empathy for child characters. In Erich Kästner's *Annaluise and Anton* (1933), if migraine is used as a device to promote sympathy, it is by suggesting child neglect from a malingering mother. Annaluise Pogge's mother is too busy theatergoing, shopping, and socializing to nurture and protect her child. The narrator inserts

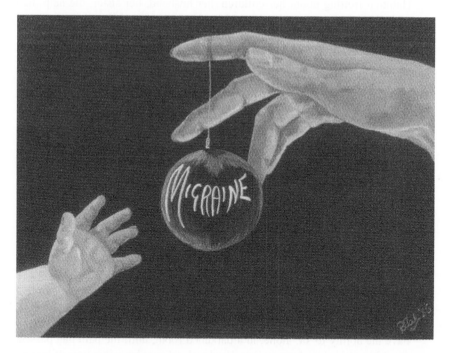

Figure 3.2 B. Clark. 1985. Migraine Art Collection. Image courtesy of Migraine Action, UK www.migraine.org.uk

moral instructions to the child reader, in case they are unclear: "She doesn't bother about her child—then why did she bring her into the world? The woman surely neglects her duty" (18). But the harshest accusations of failed mothering are found in repeated jokes about her migraine. As in the stereotype mentioned, migraine is depicted as a faked disease used as an excuse for inaction by the idle-rich mother. When Anton tells Annaluise of his own mother's occupation as a waitress, Annaluise responds, "My mother doesn't do anything. At the moment she has a headache" (26). Later, in contrast to her husband, who is always held up at work, "[h]is wife was still in her bedroom busy with her headache" (69). Frau Pogge is depicted as a thoroughly unsympathetic character, whose pain we are invited to laugh at because it is unreal: "She often suffered from this kind of headache, though her head very seldom ached" (21). The moral of the novel is clearly about parenting—that even poor little rich girls need the attention and care of their parents. The class and gender implications of idleness are always part of this explicit critique. Annaluise tells her father, "I know you have no time because you have to earn money. . . . But mother doesn't have to earn money, and yet she hasn't any time for me" (195). The mother with her fake headaches is unredeemable and unchanged in the story—instead, its primary conflict is resolved by Herr Pogge deciding to spend more time with his daughter.

If there is any suggestion that Frau Pogge's ailment is real, it is still delegiti-mized as an expression of her spoiled character, weakness, and oversensitivity. At the climax of the novel, where the "young man" of the governess breaks into their home to rob them, it is the cook who comes to the rescue. The narrator com-ments, "That deserved gratitude. And what did Frau Pogge do about it? She went to bed!" (196). The mother's response to the conflict (getting an attack of migraine) is supposed to be laughably inappropriate. She arrives after any danger has passed and all is resolved, yet she nonetheless "began to get a headache, and pulled a very agonized face," claiming "The excitement has been too much for me. . . . Please have this man taken away. He is getting terribly on my nerves" (191). Such examples speak to the pervasiveness of mother-blaming and the delegitimization of migraine in popular narratives, but the fact that they are so dominant even in a children's book also suggests that, even if we were to believe that migraine is a legitimate reason to withdraw in agony, it only affects children indirectly through their mothers, when in fact, they can inherit the disorder, and those with heredity as a factor often experience the pain at younger ages. The stereotype is not just offen-sive to women; it precludes recognizing experiences of nonwhite, working-class, or male migraineurs, and simultaneously delegitimizes child migraine even more than women's by making it seem to be out of the realm of possible consideration.

The erasure of child pain and migraine as metaphor

Child migraine is even less visible in fictional representations than in medical stud-ies and written material history, in part because of the larger cultural denial of child pain covered in my previous chapter. Even when we claim to be depicting child pain, through subtle slights, we seem to be normatizing childhood as painfree. This is particularly surprising in a literary context because of the vast tradition of utiliz-ing child illness, disability, and death as a sentimental and pathetic literary device. As Reinhard Kuhn writes, "The mortality rate among fictional children is exceed-ingly high" and yet "[t]he little victim is often less horrified by his fate than the adult who witnesses and survives his demise" (173, 193). Susan Sontag has written that "[n]ineteenth-century literature is stocked with descriptions of almost symp-tomless, unfrightened, beatific deaths . . . particularly of young people" (17). The sentimental has always been at odds with the treatment of real children by design. As Joseph Shapiro points out, "The poster child is a surefire tug at our hearts," but pity does not translate into respect, embodied knowledge, or accommodation with dignity (Shapiro 12). Where present, child pain is reduced as a literary device to the point that it becomes unthinkable in corporeal terms. Miriam Bailin writes of children in nineteenth-century fiction: "Delicate, sensitive, sickly, these characters preside over the events of the novel with a moral authority and saintliness of man-ner for which pain is both the origin and the sign" (11). When children are merely vessels of metaphoric meaning, pain becomes a disembodied symbol.

Literary child pain, then, seems to exist only to represent something else. Lois Keith demonstrates that by the mid-twentieth century, "disability and illness were mostly used as metaphors" in childhood literature (194). But, as Sontag writes,

"Illness is *not* a metaphor. . . . [T]he most truthful way of regarding illness—and the healthiest way of being ill—is one most purified of, most resistant to, metaphoric thinking" (3). Sontag is being hyperbolic, not facile, in suggesting this impossible resistance to the potentially dishonest impulses and couched biases of metaphor—she is expressing the offensiveness of certain metaphors to real, subjectively situated, experience. Pain is *not* a metaphor to those in it. While many will contest that metaphor allows us to imaginatively get into the minds of others and increase empathy, metaphor is also a dangerous reinterpretation that can limit our perception just as much as it opens it.

Frustrating attempts to make pain more visible is the fact that we are in denial about our denial. Even our interdisciplinary attempts to acknowledge the limits of the discursive often mislead us into projecting without check. In *Pain and Its Transformations: The Interface of Biology and Culture*, which by its title suggests a genuine effort to bridge discourses from multiple disciplines in discussions of pain, Elaine Scarry felt it necessary to preface her contribution with this admonition:

> Like most of you, I see pain as underscoring the connection between "body" and world. But I also want to insist on a slightly more restricted sense of pain, limited to the physical. Many of you talk about suffering, grief, or depression as pain, and I recognize the accuracy of that and salute it. But I think that on some levels physical pain is distinguishable from these other things.
>
> (2007, 64)

And indeed, it is distinguishable in necessary ways.

Of course, suffering, and even what we call pain, always has a psychological and emotional dimension that can't be dismissed (it's simply beyond the scope of this book). Any inexplicable suffering (like depression) has the senseless word-destroying quality attributed to pain, and for that reason invites the analogy. As David T. Mitchell and Sharon L. Snyder have argued in *Narrative Prosthesis*, "The corporeal metaphor offers narrative the one thing it cannot possess—an anchor in materiality. Such a process embodies the materiality of metaphor" (63). When someone, through a literary flourish, describes *ennui* as pain it physicalizes an even more linguistically elusive state. But when scholars lump all sorts of suffering under the umbrella term "pain studies," then proceed to incorporate any emotional state from feeling suicidal to boredom, grave misunderstandings can occur, and the very empathy and understanding we promote will be offensive to some and ineffectual to others. Such approaches have broadened the definition of their subject beyond any precise application.

Much of the resulting disconnect is caused by disciplinary baggage:

> We have centuries of literature that has profound expressiveness for romantic heartache, for horrible forms of psychotic pain, and so forth, but the number of works expressing the brute fact of cancer pain, burn pain, extreme headache, et cetera, would probably fit in an ordinary binder.
>
> (Scarry 2007, 64)

As a literary scholar, I can't resist in this book, for example, using my own meta-phors and those of others (analogies with war/weapons, scars/healing, and runts/nonhuman animals). Each of these analogies comes with a risk that I will belittle one position by comparing it with another, yet I keep them hoping that together they will convey a unique perspective of young embodied invisible impairment that has been shared with me by many others in figurative ways. Even the primary subversive strategy of "visibility" projects hinges upon a figure that is exclusion-ary in privileging sightedness. In 1963 Erving Goffman warned that "perceptibil-ity" or "evidentness" would be more inclusive, accurate terms for expressing the same goals (48), but now that the tactics of "visibility" politics have evolved so intertwined with visual culture in an age of visual literacy, the term seems to be sticking.

When we must limit ourselves to the discursive we are even more trapped by the solipsism of metaphor. This has been demonstrated time and again to me when I'm asked what I've been working on and tell fellow literary scholars "child migraine." I've often heard variations of "sounds like a headache!" or even the mystifying "what an important metaphor." Most assume that I'm looking at such a topic solely in a figurative manner simply because in literature we are surrounded by a buffer through which everything is discursive. But pain is not simply discursive to me. It hurts. And sometimes, so do metaphors. Melanie Thernstrom has a similar reac-tion to religious idealizations of pain: "The idea of pain as spiritual transformation offends me. It seems, in a word, perverse" (69). She and I are both responding on a personalized level to a language problem that has long been discussed by disability theorists and resulted in a complicated and precarious "policing" of metaphor that is very challenging to keep up with. Stephen Loftus has described this process: "The issue is not *whether* to use metaphors, but *which* metaphors to use" (218). This process can become so linguistically self-conscious that it halts discourse (I, for example, was just about to say it "paralyzes" discourse, indicating how difficult it is, from one's own limited subjectivity, to avoid figurations that are insensitive to others even while discussing that very act). Amy Vidali advises against simply reacting at the intersection where "discursive construction meets embodied reality" to "go beyond 'policing' language" (33–34). We have to recognize our subjective situatedness, not necessarily advocate an ever-increasingly complex "policing of metaphors" for experience. Sami Schalk provides a practical middle ground: "be responsible" and "be accountable and open to criticism" (17). Certainly, in the precarious identity politics of disability, voicing diverse perspectives is just the start; we have to go beyond listening into practice. And our words must be taken as fluid invitations to constant revision.

Metaphors can serve to legitimate impaired experience or permit its erasure. In my next two chapters I collect migraineur expressions that will allow, I hope, the former process. In terms of being aware, however, of the latter consequences, there are questions we can ask about what linguistic work our analogies are doing. Mel Y. Chen proposes (via Lennard Davis) that we look at linguistic repercussions. Do the potential ends justify expressive means? If our language relies upon analogies that are objectifying or dehumanizing, they can clearly be used toward nefarious results (2012, 41–43). Chen uses Terri Schiavo's 13-day death by starvation and dehydration as a good example. Redefined by her "vegetative" state as "a vegetable," she was both objectified and dehumanized, thus enabling a painful death in the name of ending "pain" for which there was no evidence. A cautionary tale in the slippery stakes of language and disability, I find Chen's criteria enlightening in the case of representing children with migraine. Child migraineurs, where represented, are typically objectified, and their pain is conveniently erased from consideration just as easily as pain can be misprojected upon others who are nonverbally painfree. As I have periodically hinted, children are often dehumanized in anthropocentric discourse through lumping scientific and literary comparisons with nonhuman animals, though ultimately I will argue that this secondary tendency can also bridge understandings if met with a willingness to recognize human animality and vulnerability.

If language is dangerously full of slippage in the discourse surrounding both disability and children, it nevertheless is a rich and necessary avenue for accessing greater compassion, especially as both subjects are so complexly and opaquely constructed. Stuart Murray writes, in his study of autism, that when we ask political questions about the representation of neurologically atypical experience, they are "more cultural than neurological" (64). Murray's analysis provides penetrating opportunities for insight into migraine as well, through both telling contrasts and even more surprising similarities. Autism, a condition that affects males more than females (at a ratio of 4 to 1), is typically depicted as masculine in popular culture and even as resulting from what has been depicted as an "extreme male brain" by Hans Asperger in 1944 and Simon Baron-Cohen as late as 2003 (Murray 155). As with feminized migraine, rampant generalizing is to some degree a result of a gendered predominance in diagnosis. Murray traces the discursive gendering of autism just as sociologist Joanna Kempner has migraine (their books make an excellent pairing for anyone interested in genderings of disability). More germane to my point here, however, is the curious age-typing Murray considers:

> Pervasive and present, autism is not something one grows out of. And yet, given that this is the case, contemporary cultural fascination with autism nevertheless relentlessly focuses on the figure of the child when seeking to explore what autism is and what it might mean. . . . Even though it is obvious that children with autism will become adults with autism, the sense that the condition somehow affects children *more* than adults is itself pervasive.
>
> (139)

As with the misperception that "the migraineur" is by definition adult, the faulty presumption that a person with autism is always a child demands a cultural explanation. Both generalizations about age are so inaccurate that they raise philosophical questions that could lead to tomes of study and speculation. Why do cultural productions so narrowly present the person with autism as a child and the person with migraine as an adult? Stuart Murray suggests the sentimental power of poster children in fund-raising or the profiting "treatment" industry as possible motives for the rhetorical aging down of autism (140). Patrick McDonagh's book in the same series provides evidence that could also suggest projecting narratives of mythical innocence or casting out as changelings in cases of intellectual difference, which seems consistent with American tendencies to rigidly classify struggling children as "Mad, Bad, Sad, or Can't Add" (McDonagh 4, 11 and Woodhouse 280). In contrast, there seem to be no ready categories in which to place a child with migraine. Rather than combating offensive *mis*representations, it appears that child migraineurs struggle to be represented at all. Ultimately, as concerns autism, Stuart Murray suggests that the best explanation is that "the concentration on autism is . . . a particular and peculiar *adult* concern. It is driven by a generation of adults, many of whom see autism as a contemporary epidemic that threatens their children" (141). And, indeed, this is a telling common factor reproduced in stereotypes of autism and migraine—both are continually represented in terms of how they affect parents or parenting. Such unexpected, crucial insights come from considering the intersectionality of ageism and ableism, rather than isolating analysis of separate identity experiences across an individual's lifespan.

A related insight can be found in a wealth of recent scholarship on temporality. Age creep (up or down) in representations of disability is a consequence of norming in part because it is so effectively overlooked. Linear developmentalism underlies Western constructions of childhood so completely that their biases and temporal constructedness often goes undetected. In his essay "In Any Event: Moving Rhizomatically in Peter Cameron's *Someday This Pain Will Be Useful to You*," and elsewhere in his work, childhood studies scholar Markus Bohlmann argues that we should radically destabilize our rhetorically sedimented, static temporalizing of childhood. Using Deleuze and Guattari's analogy of arborescent versus rhizomatic *growth*, Bohlmann encourages uprooting the temporal confinement of the teleology of development that favors adulthood as the positive end that justifies oppressive means, which might be effectively countered by "departing from the vocabulary of growth and instead implementing words and modes of rhizomatic movement as a nonteleological alternative" (386). Such a perspective particularly illuminates the case of Ashley X, whose medical treatment has been of great interest in disability politics, and is equally revealing about the politics of childhood.

The child known as Ashley X was born in 1997 and diagnosed with "static encephalopathy" shortly thereafter. The medical consensus was that she would never be able to move autonomously or gain a capacity for speech as she physically developed over time. Demonstrating the fondness for linear, temporal absolutes so integral to and unquestioned in American approaches toward children, the media repeatedly reported that she would cognitively arrest development with the "brain of a 6-month old."[20] Fearing that as she grew in size her care would be too difficult to manage, and under the advisement of a medical team, Ashley's parents decided to stunt her growth and prevent the bodily changes of puberty through aggressive hormonal treatment and surgical removal of her breast buds and reproductive organs. Tobin Siebers has explained that "[a]t the heart of the controversy is the question of whether Ashley's parents are rescuing their daughter from pain or abusing her, but pain remains in either case the deciding factor" (2010, 185). As with the case of Terri Schiavo, Siebers uses the case of Ashley X to demonstrate "both the association of pain with disability and how pain takes on contradictory guises to serve different ends" (2010, 188). In the context of the U.S. history of under-treating child pain, Ashley's "treatment" particularly speaks to how arbitrarily and conveniently our shifting rhetoric can be made to serve inconsistent purposes for and by adults. Procedures some have called "barbaric" were justified in accounts by the logic that they would spare Ashley from menstrual cramps and the discomfort of support straps if she inherited the large breasts that run in her family. Ashley X's experience is concrete proof of the discursive power to inflict pain (even in the name of alleviating pain) on a child patient—to deny or inflict it according to adult needs. Like many confined to nonconsent by lack of ability to communicate, Ashley X was redefined through diagnosis, parental decisions, medical technology, *and* language—she would become famous as her parents' "pillow angel."

I bring up this lengthy digression on such a profound and controversial case to indicate an extreme and harsh example of how necessary and concretely irrefutable the seemingly abstract and theoretical project of Bohlmann's "departing from the vocabulary of growth" actually is for and in the embodied reality of young persons. His argument complements queer/crip feminist Alison Kafer's in-depth analysis of the Ashley X case in *Feminist Queer Crip* (2013). Kafer writes,

> As becomes clear in both the parental and medical justifications of the Treatment, the case of Ashley X offers a stark illustration of how disability is often understood as a kind of disruption in the temporal field. Supporters of the Treatment frame Ashley's disability as a kind of temporal disjuncture; not only had she failed to grow and develop "normally," but her mind and body were developing at different speeds from each other.
>
> (48)

Rather than permitting her to become a "baby in an adult's body," her carers arrested "the present Ashley in time" as "an eternal child," literally infantilizing her (53, 48, 49). It is just astounding enough to know that this is *medically possible* that it might be easy to miss the subtler implications of Kafer's connecting insight: "In this desire for mind and body to align, what we see is a temporal framing of disability dovetailing with a developmental model of childhood" (53). It is the diagnosis of Ashley's "6-month-old's brain" and her "infant-like dependency and passivity," not her size, that made her medical interventions *rhetorically possible*.

Tobin Siebers warns against assuming that the body of a visibly impaired person is a body in pain, and the reverse holds true: we cannot assume that a person is painfree simply because we cannot see their pain. Further complicating childhood disability, however, is a persistent adult desire, and resulting denial, that allows us to imagine development as a natural progression in which we only gradually accrue capacity for pain. By halting Ashley's development, her carers may be able to better protect her, but by freezing her in "eternal childhood," they also make it easier for us to imagine her painfree. And if we hold onto adult-serving sentimentality about tiny bodies being impervious to "grown-up" pain, we are capable of barbarous treatment in spite of the best of intentions.

Though fictional kids with head pain hardly register as dramatic subject matter in comparison to profound interventions like those previously described, they are likewise equally malleable through our "vocabularies of growth" and worthy of similar analysis. The prejudicial force of literary representations can, as Stuart Murray says, "offer ideas of cure by stealth" or allow us to imagine those in pain as pain-free quite subtly (211). Such narratives demand counternarratives. Like some of the adult migraineurs depicted in the film and novels already mentioned in this chapter, fictional child migraineurs are not cast in a legitimating light, if at all, though I did find one exception. A rare example that centers on a child character (though initially through her retrospective as an adult), and provides a legitimating counterstory to those of Maxi's mother and Bernice Pritchard, is Moufida Tlatli's film *The Silences of the Palace* (1994). Set in a wealthy Tunisian household in 1956, the film follows the memories of its protagonist, Alia, while she is migraining in the middle of her own conflicted adulthood (as the mistress of a man who will not marry her because of class differences, and who has just asked her to have an abortion). Her flashbacks are directly related to the migraine attack framing the film—she is recognizing that although she escaped the abusive traps of her mother's life, she is experiencing, nonetheless, similar insurmountable challenges. Like the examples previously shown, these challenges generally reflect upon motherhood. As with *Fortunata*'s Maxi, Alia's migraines have been loosely connected to her being an illegitimate child, though in this case we see the mother in a completely sympathetic light—she has no options, no choice, because she is a domestic and sexual servant in what looks like an authentic, not Orientalized, version of a harem (reminiscent of Fatima Mernissi's nonfictional *Dreams of Trespass: Tales of a Harem Childhood*, the women and children are isolated in a gated residence). Like Emily Tallis, though in a much more class-determined and substantial way, Alia's mother, Khedija, is unable to adequately nurture her daughter, and like Bernice Pritchard, Khedija is raped, but this case we see through the eyes of a sympathetic daughter. Anne Donadey has written of the film: "Such an ambivalent and unspoken situation makes it even more difficult for Alia to deal with her parents' relationship and for Khedija to protect herself and her daughter from incestuous sexual predation" (40). And, in an even rarer model, this film acknowledges the child migraineur by showing these events through her perspective.

As with *That Beautiful Somewhere,* the opening conflict of the film is an attack triggered during a public performance, the migraine a device, but one full of meaning:

> Physical symptoms such as chronic migraines, fainting, and dissociation recur in Alia as part of the film's representation of gender and sexual trauma. At the beginning of the film, Alia is shown having a long-lasting migraine. . . . [H]er migraines begin not with her witnessing Bechir raping her mother (when we also see her rubbing her temples), but her moving from child to adolescent and therefore her entry into a world in which she will be targeted sexually in the same way her mother has been.

> (40)

Such a dramatization equates migraine not with idle luxury or malingering but with trauma, which is a legitimate factor rather than stereotyped dismissal. In fact, Tlatli uses migraine as a framing stance from which to critique the vicious structural inequities that trap women into everyday trauma: "Alia's migraines are connected to women's gender and sexuality, which are lived in the mode of trauma and violence and whose sexual abuse is repeatedly swallowed through silences" (40–41). Silence again. Whereas Bernice Pritchard silences her own screams with a pillow to be a darling for her family, this film in contrast invites us to view the silencing as yet another symptom of trigemony's oppression.

Unfortunately, however, *The Silences of the Palace* is one of the only legitimating narratives I could find focalized through the perspective of a fictional child migraineur. It is curious that the two most legitimating fictional examples I've found come from film while all the stereotyping and dismissal originally appears in literature. Possibly the visual dimension makes erasure of pain more difficult, which is certainly a premise of visibility projects. In contrast (but consistent with the historical patterns I discussed in chapter 2), the literary figuration of children in pain is almost always objectifying. We do not usually see a child with migraine or even a child in pain as a subject, especially in a legitimating narrative focalized through their experience. Instead they serve as objects, to reflect the metaphorical "pain" of others, or at least their migraine performs it.

The fiction of faking

Like cultural age-profiling of impairments, the performance of migraine through fictional children usually brings the focus back either compassionately or judgmentally on a caretaker rather than the child. *Triggered* (2013), a YA novel by Vicki Grant, epitomizes this problem. The book focuses on the dwindling romance of two teenagers, Jade and Mick, the conflict between whom is dramatized through the migraines of Jade's four-year-old brother, Gavin. Chapters alternate point of view through the teenaged characters, ostensibly focused on Gavin's condition but never focalized through his perspective. Instead, Jade emotionally manipulates Mick in response to Gavin's attacks. Although the slim book is filled with details that might inform an unfamiliar reader with the experience and challenges of managing child migraine (dietary restrictions, scintillating scotoma, vomiting, trips home early from day care, the need for stillness, quiet, and dark), Gavin is merely a device for dramatizing how punishing psychological manipulation can become; he is an object of his sister's mental disorder. It is clear he can serve as an object because he is a young child with a condition that's undetectable without articulate report: "He's such a brave little guy because of all the pain he's endured. Sometimes it's hard to know when he's actually hurt" (51). Many descriptions hinge on this impossibility of comprehending child migraine or legitimately proving it: "He's four years old. You think a four-year-old can make himself throw up? Go pale?" (67). The conflict of the book hinges on a delegitimized diagnosis: "Even the doctors don't do much good" and migraines are "painful but not serious. Kids get them all the time" (70, 86). The only moment of agency the child has in the book is calling out his sister in a lie that reveals she has been purposely giving him MSG to trigger his attacks to manipulate her boyfriend (112). She has Munchausen's and he is her proxy.

What bothers me about the story is the unspoken hint throughout that two teenagers are overreacting to simple headaches. This is the assumption that is supposed to make obvious (and it *is* obvious) that something is wrong here. Not Gavin's headaches but Jade's reactions. Unfortunately, migraine is just the kind of disorder that is expedient for demonstrating such a dynamic. If she caused a lethal illness the book would be too serious, and we'd have to invest so much empathy for the child character that we couldn't concentrate on the silly but twisted "romantic" elements of the novel. Just as body metaphors "anchor" a fictional experience in materiality, child pain easily represents another's implicitly far more serious problem, invoking not sympathy for the younger figure but attention on another (think of the formula films in which a child is kidnapped and the audience is expected to see this solely as the parents' emotional drama).

In this case we learn about the "secondary gains" that lead to "pain behavior," so often attributed to children, in the teenaged Jade. And so her disorder, Munchausen's, has its roots in early discoveries that she has gotten from attention from pain: "I burned myself before. I remember how much it hurt. It was right before Dad left. He put this special ointment on it and let me stay up late watching TV with him. I was only seven, but the scar's still there" (81–82). Is the flip side of this message that we shouldn't take child pain too seriously? That we might be encouraging young malingerers? And if we are even more prone to believing that a young person will lie for attention, migraine is easy to fake and so even less believable coming from a demographic we're so easily convinced is simply lying. Marc Feldman, an expert on factitious disorders, cites a pertinent example of a 15-year old, "Chris," who posed as a migraineur on a Usenet group:

> His reports about his struggle with intractable migraines were moving, particularly in view of his youth and the unique personal qualities he described. Over time, Chris disclosed that he also suffered with hemophilia as well as a seizure disorder due to abusive head trauma his estranged father had inflicted. Despite these ailments and his brother's recent death from AIDS, he was performing superbly as a fourth-year medical student.
>
> (Feldman 163)

As the implausibilities mounted, fellow posters started to question his honesty, but a telling detail was too hard to believe: "[I]t strained credulity that Chris played the drums even in the throes of a migraine" (164). Migraine seems to have been Chris's gateway lie—convincing only up to a point. But the fact that he gained the temporary trust of others with migraine speaks to how easily it is faked, which only disserves those who truly suffer from an already difficult-to-prove condition.

Child migraine, because it is presumed too nonexistent or trifling to justify genuine anxiety or concern, becomes the perfect "disorder" to express nervous over-concern on the part of a caretaker. In Mike Albo's fictionalized memoir *Hornito,*

My Lie Life (2000), in order to indicate an idealized yet hypernormalized suburban childhood, Albo writes,

> My mom wipes the counter with a damp rag and says for me to drink a glass of water. It was one of her quicker decisions, because there has been a spate of newscasts on local television about child migraines. We go to a doctor who wears a tie with Bugs Bunny on it and he sticks his cold ear otoscope in my ear and it feels good. Nothing is wrong.
>
> (45)

Migraine, so easily perceived as an imaginary ailment, is a particularly pertinent condition to discussing liminal diagnosis on the body-mind continuum, as Carla Cantor explains, "The medical gray area that exists between the body and brain has created a vast diagnostic vacuum," in which migraine is easily ignored or demarginalized (152). In fact, it is as difficult to disprove as it is to prove, making it a common choice of official diagnosis by doctors trying to legitimate hypochondria for insurance[21] purposes (155).

So it is not just in fiction that children can be objects in performing migraine as a fiction itself. In Julie Gregory's *Sickened: The Memoir of a Munchausen by Proxy Childhood*, migraine also provides her mother with the gateway lie. Migraine is the fallback illness she goes to when more alarming or easily disproven conditions are dismissed by doctors, who nonetheless seem strangely willing to liberally prescribe migraine away, especially because of the mother's persistence (perhaps out of frustration, even). As Julie is still young enough to be wondering "What is a headache, *exactly*?" her mother and doctor are already reasoning through to a diagnosis of migraine and prescription of Ergostat (ergotamine), rather quickly compared to the run-around and reticence toward diagnosing children with migraine that was the norm in the 1970s (26–27). And such performances have a real effect in delegitimizing the disease, not just to the general public but even more consequentially to doctors they depend upon for treatment. Joanna Kempner cites multiple studies showing that even though headache is the most common complaint neurologists see in patients, it is the least covered disorder in their training (56); that doctors find headache patients "time consuming," "more emotionally draining," and "having more psychiatric problems" than other patients (8); and that a quarter of neurologists in one survey agreed that "[m]any headache patients have motivation to maintain their disability" (55). Malingerers, fictional and real, do not help reduce the legitimacy deficit and put an even greater burden of proof on actual migraineurs to get the help or accommodations they need. And this makes migraineurs defensively cling to the biology of the brain, the disease model, and even the success of their abortive medications as proof that their illness is not made in their own minds, which is unfortunate, because dealing with intractable migraine—that cannot be resolved with quick fixes—requires integrating the body-mind to unleash the power of our minds to help us cope with breakthrough pain.

Though historically some children have had access to the earlier treatments mentioned in this chapter—trepanation, opiates, ergot—for the most part that access is limited due to practical considerations of greater dangers to their health. The therapeutic orphaning of child migraineurs is slowly decreasing due to pharmacological investments in making sure triptans are safe enough for juvenile use, but the youngest migraineurs will most likely always need to be excluded, and unless we have greater industry oversight, any choices they have will be determined by a profit-driven market, thus requiring intensive consumer education. During the 1990s, the "decade of the brain," neurology turned hyperspecialized attention to migraine after triptans proved what a lucrative, captive market the headache industry could supply. Riding the crest of the triptan wave was the rise of prophylactic medications (especially anticonvulsants), often prescribed off-label in trial-and-error style,[22] which sometimes has made guinea pigs out of children—a demographic left out of many medical trials to, ironically, protect them.

One of the migraineurs I interviewed brings an interesting individual perspective to these historic developments. Carrie Hall, whose migraine attacks began when she was 11 years old (her brother's began at age 7), grew up as a teen in the 1980s with a neurologist as her father. In the pre-triptan days she and her brother tried many prescription medications to no effect. In an effort to discourage pain behavior, Carrie's parents required her to attend school on migraine days, trying to medicate and make it through. She says of the pre-triptan decade, "I was drugged out of my skull" (pre-triptan abortives, like Fiorinal or Esgic, were comprised of caffeine, an anti-inflammatory, and barbiturates). She is direct about the personal cost-benefit analysis she did once she found something that worked (Neurontin): "I don't care if I'm spacy, at least I am not as incoherent as I am in pain," and "[I]f it takes ten years of my life, fine." This was not careless bargaining but a long process of negotiating risks and finding boundaries: "even Mr. Take-a-Pill-for-It [her father] said 'Don't take Depakote.'" And never narcotics, as "they only made it worse." Neurology in the Age of the Brain was a pharmaceutical game. Now Carrie is very outspoken about the experience, but she can remember being young and internalizing an awareness of the lack of patience, empathy, or even belief others had for her condition: "Growing up with chronic pain that has no relief, you just have to pretend you're not in pain and go along with your day . . . I learned to hide being in pain and might have learned that too well." Children need other options than silence.

For the most part children have the fewest and least aggressive options for managing migraine attacks, like guided imagery, self-distraction, elimination diets, relaxation therapy, acupuncture, and biofeedback. Unfortunately, nondrug options are less funded for patients and not subsidized for development; as C. M. Shifflett pithily puts it,

> There is no multi-billion-dollar international biofeedback cartel. Doctors don't get trips to Hawaii as reward for prescribing hand-warming. No one hires mega-buck advertising firms to ghostwrite phony research articles to place in medical journals, nor do they have the money to bribe MDs to sign off on them as pharmaceutical companies have done.

(258)

And so these methods are even less available to children who desperately could use them. But the reality is that they should be made available to all. And they are usually cost-efficient and riskless methods that, even after a few sessions, can be used for the rest of one's life by putting the mind more in tune with autonomic responses. M. Carlean Gilbert found that child migraineurs who are granted autonomy, have reasonable control over their medications, view themselves as healthy, and have access to a larger support network in which they are free to communicate concerns, are more likely to cope effectively in a lasting manner (297–284). Child advocate and law professor Ursula Kilkelly has demonstrated in multiple studies the importance of child participation and being heard in the medical context (2011, 2012). With Bensted et al., Kilkelly concluded in 2014, from 2,023 completed surveys from eight European countries, that young patients report the following priorities: "The most important item for all age groups was being listened to. Children rated pain control and the presence of parents more important than either understanding the doctor or being able to ask questions. . . . Being listened to is the most important priority at all ages" (Bensted 160). Children can be ideal copers if given the right circumstances. Being silenced and controlled must give way to being heard and gaining a sense of control.

Real children, far from being the empty vessels of signification we see in fiction, are actually model copers in training the mind to work with the body in overcoming (or, more realistically in the case of migraine, coping with) pain. They are far more adaptive than adults at alternative therapies. In contrast to their literary counterparts, real children take control when taught coping techniques and can become the active agents of their treatment. One 11-year-old migraineur described the coping strategy he developed after guided imagery sessions, which combines relaxation techniques with distraction:

> I lie down and then I let myself go all over like I'm the laundry bag emptied on the bed, you know? Like all over. Then I start right at the beginning of the game (baseball) against (rival school) and it's not just a shut-out, it's like a real massacre, the whole nine innings we do everything great and I hit a homer.
>
> (quoted in McGrath 2001, 133)

This child migraineur is the subject of his distraction fantasy, not the object of a victim narrative. Learning to relax rather than brace against pain prepares young migraineurs for future attacks, and in some cases may even provide life skills that lower stress and the number of attacks.

Children are more fluid than adults at grasping mental control over otherwise involuntary bodily experience, especially through visualization. This is because they are still learning the tricks our perceptions can play, as indicated by a 2013 study on the "rubber-hand illusion," in which children were shown to be more responsive to imagining a rubber hand as their own (Cowie et al. 2013). Emergent body sense is important to self-protection and highly dependent on visual cues, but keeping that body sense open might also have health benefits—for example, phantom limb pain has been successfully reduced in some cases with mirrors and visual illusion (Ramachandran 2011). Utilizing this flexible body sense, biofeedback (and now neurobiofeedback) connects technological indicators of the child's vitals so that the patient can practice relaxing and see or hear her or his body's immediate response, redirect cranial blood flow back to extremities, strengthening awareness of the mind-body connection, the power of the mind to train the body, and the power of the body to learn, remember, and more easily revisit relaxed states reached through guided practice. Such therapies do not necessarily lessen pain, but they become tools that will help young migraineurs cope. The young person in pain who is able to imagine himself limp like a laundry bag or tickled by a paintbrush on her prosthetic hand is modeling both an integrated bodymind *and* mentally transcending the body's experience at the same time.

Elizabeth Grosz has argued that

> the body provides a point of mediation between what is perceived as purely internal and accessible only to the subject and what is external and publicly observable, a point from which to rethink the opposition between the inside and the outside.
>
> (57)

Biofeedback connects the inside and outside, demonstrating that "killing the mind" and being at war with our bodies aren't the only models—some relief can be found in strengthening their connection. Guided imagery and distraction techniques, on the other hand, require that you imaginatively sever that connection—mind over matter. Likewise, the literature of the mind and the material history of the body have been telling very different stories about migraine. To get a more holistic understanding we have to be willing to consider diverse, even contradictory, voicings and visions.

Though literary migraine can familiarize readers with diagnostic detail and concrete hints of a sometimes desperate material history of treatments, it also obscures pain in romanticized portrayals of aura and victim-blaming rhetoric. Firsthand accounts reveal a more complicated collective range of experience that needs to be amplified. In my next chapter I will rely more heavily on the direct reports of authentic migraineurs to continue delving, from the inside, into the discursive practices and stereotypes they must resist in their efforts to be seen and heard.

Notes

1 I recommend listening to the Live Room version: www.youtube.com/watch?v=W29uD5Gf5Fc.
2 In *The Body in Pain*, Elaine Scarry refers to how "pain causes a reversion to the pre-language of cries and groans" (6). I connect these sounds to nonhuman expressions not to dehumanize but to emphasize that pain makes us aware of the vulnerability of our animal bodies.
3 Term coined by Perry Davis for his own recipe in 1845 (see McTavish 32–34).
4 In the U.S. context, especially due to the Harrison Narcotic Act of 1914.
5 The exact number is 4.43 times (Breslau et al. 723).

6   James C. Wilson and Cynthia Lewiecki-Wilson point out that even the language of the 1990 Americans with Disabilities Act promotes a continued conceptual split of the bodymind because "its language, 'physical or mental,' reinforces the separation of mind and body even as contemporary neuroscience rejects such dualistic models" (10).

7   Antonio R. Damasio writes, "More may have been learned about the brain and the mind in the 1990s – the so-called decade of the brain – than during the entire previous history of psychology and neuroscience" (112).

8   Migraine history includes the famous migraine that Grant had when Lee surrendered (ending Grant's attack) and the attack that Aaron Burr had during a consequential meeting with fellow-migraineur Thomas Jefferson (see Fleming). But migraine history could also be written to include less recognized migraineurs like Virginia Reed's mother from the Donner Party. I'm not sure if the fact these compensatory lists tend to highlight more men than women is a function of the sexism of history (that more prominent personalities are male) or sexism on the part of those who compile them (finding male figures more legitimating). I like to bring up Elvis as an example of someone, like others mentioned here, whose addiction and drug abuse probably began in an effort to control migraine pain. The general public tends to only know that he was an addict, not that he was a migraineur. One of my colleagues jokingly calls the baggie with migraine meds I keep in my book bag my "Elvis baggie." Little did she know, at first, how aptly applied the term was. It stuck.

9   I include both *Alice* books in my analysis, though the first is usually emphasized in such readings. By the logic of diagnostic criticism, the Red Queen's rushing to stay in place could arguably be a representation of the aura called "the rushes," though I don't believe I've seen the argument in print.

10   Michael Roos writes that "there are two songs which draw virtually their entire meaning from images found in the Alice books, 'Lucy in the Sky with Diamonds' and 'I Am the Walrus,' songs which cannot be fully understood without some knowledge of Lewis Carroll" (20).

11   Stuart Murray writes, "Retrospective diagnosis is . . . a fraught process that is all too open to the abuse of the lazy claim, but it can also be a radical critical intervention that is enlightening in extending the parameters of how we understand and read disability" (51). When I told neurologist Joost Haan that child migraineurs were unrepresented in literature he advised, "They are probably there, you just have to look with the right eyes" (personal interview). Certainly Stuart Murray's method in *Representing Autism: Culture, Narrative, Fascination* demonstrates how a scholar can "diagnose" historical figures and fictional characters while balancing speculation very effectively with rigor.

12   Though LSD was first produced in 1938, Hofmann would not discover its psychotropic properties until 1943 (Hofmann 4, 14). Ergot was isolated and thus controllable for relatively safe prescription use in 1918 (4), and predominated in the abortive treatment of migraine from then until the introduction of triptans in the late 1980s and early '90s.

13   Ergot poisoning could infect entire communities through the ingestion of bread made with rye during wet seasons, with terrible effects, including psychosis, St. Anthony's fire (perceived burning of the limbs), and death (see Matossian). Often ergotism resulted in blackening of the fingers and toes, represented in many paintings and eerily familiar to the much milder symptom, Raynaud's syndrome, which migraineurs often experience.

14   For more on Edward Woakes's report on ergot in 1868, see Koehler and Isler (2002).

15   It is said the same happened to Charles Darwin (Friedman 668), an interesting parallel only in that both – one fictional, one real – are pleasing departures from the cliché feminized excuse "not tonight" that Joanna Kempner documents so well.

16   Laudanum was commonly used for migraine, but Galdós presents it as a last resort: "Maxi's condition didn't improve, which made it necessary to resort to the extreme: laudanum. The patient himself asked for it from between the sheets in whimpers so faint they didn't seem to fit the magnitude of the bed. Fortunata picked up the eyedropper and . . . [i]nstead of six drops she added only five" (394). To put this dosage in context, Samuel Taylor Coleridge took 20,000 drops per week at the height of his addiction (Booth, 44).

Coleridge's use of laudanum began at age eight (42). Before regulation, children were given laudanum, "calming cordial for infants," and soothing opiates (58, 64).

17 Steinbeck's wife, Elaine Steinbeck, highlighted a preoccupation with illness as one result of the author's unhealthy early years: "It wouldn't be wrong to say that John was a hypochondriac. . . . He was always worrying about being sick, treating himself very gingerly" (Parini 20). His biographer writes that Steinbeck's childhood illness "seems to have given him a sense of himself as someone on the edge of life, someone vulnerable – physically and emotionally" (20).

18 In the film adaptation also titled *The Wayward Bus* (1957), the depiction of Mrs. Pritchard is even less flattering. She is shown as a psychobabbling hypochondriac, a privileged, frigid faddist (not really a person with migraine at all), thus even more delegitimating of migraine implicitly for the viewer who knows the original narrative and medicalized identity inspiring the representation. An even more vilifying depiction of migraine occurs in another 1950's film adaptation, *The Caine Mutiny* (1954). Captain Queeg's migraine is repeatedly used as evidence of his instability in order to justify mutiny (see Kramer).

19 Jeannette Stirling writes of the classist bias in discourse from the 1890s differentiating migraine from epilepsy, two conditions that throughout most of modern medical history have been considered closely related in physical cause, though socially constructed in dramatically diverging ways: "[M]igraine and epilepsy necessarily belonged to different classes of persons. . . . Headache in this scenario is associated with the highly strung and evolved nervous system, whereas associations between epilepsy and the 'dull and stupid' necessarily preclude the epileptic from experiencing pain in 'his' head" (41).

20 My summary of this case heavily paraphrases Siebers (2010) and Kafer (2013).

21 Cantor writes, "[H]ypochondria, for insurance purposes, is listed as disorder number 300.7 in diagnostic manuals. Ironically, it is not likely to be covered by most insurance plans, so to make [it] diagnostically acceptable, doctors usually describe the problem on health forms as irritable bowel syndrome, migraine, or allergic sensitivity – whichever physical symptoms predominate. But this is confusing. Aren't IBS and migraine mind-body diagnoses?" (155).

22 For details on this situation, see Loder and Biondi (2004), Hampton (2007), and Yao (2013). Neurontin has a particularly interesting history, in that it was fraudulently advertised for migraine prophylaxis.

4   Testifying against trigemony

F u trigeminal nerve. Making life hell . . .

Jason G, online comment

According to biographer Curtis Cate, Friedrich Nietzsche's migraines became particularly troublesome in his thirteenth year, making him "permanently unwell" (13, 184). He spent much time in his boarding school's "sickroom," and attacks seem to have been prompted by weather, schoolwork, exams, and his intensive independent intellectual exercise. In fact, one of his doctors recommended, "Be more stupid and you will feel better" (Cate 184). Against this advice, unfortunately for his health but fortunately for us, Nietzsche obsessively studied and produced in spite of his pain, which clearly affected his worldview. At age 16, Nietzsche could have been just as easily speaking of migraine as of fate, in fact as a migraineur he seems to have intertwined the two,[1] when he said,

> What is it that pulls the soul of so many men of power down to the commonplace, thereby hindering a higher flight of ideas? A fatalistic structure of skull and spine; the condition and nature of their parents. . . . We have been influenced. And we lack the strength to react against this influence or even to recognize that we have been influenced. It is a painful feeling to have given up one's independence through an unconscious acceptance of external impressions, stifling the capacity of the soul . . . and enduring the planting of the seeds of abberations [*sic*] within the soul and against the will.
>
> ("Fate and History: Thoughts,"14)

Restraints against free will, visible and invisible, become communicated as biologically fatalistic—as unnegotiable as "skull and spine." Our biology is sometimes ideologically inflected as fate (or ideology is inflected biologically as fate), depicted as essential rather than personally mutable. Of course on one level Nietzsche is talking about what we now describe as environmental factors or social construction, but he does so with the language of a stark and unyielding physicality, with a wry awareness of the deterministic manner in which ideology, too, can be so difficult to change, seemingly to prevail as fate, through the consensus-making of hegemony. Likewise, migraine can prevail in the meanest and most banal manner—against our efforts to prevent or abort attacks, just as hegemonic forces can determine who will suffer more or who will get relief.

One could argue that migraine is just a fact of "skull and spine," or as we now more precisely understand, the central and peripheral nervous systems. In the twenty-first century, the biological "forces" behind the attacks are more concretely, though not fully, understood. Scott Fishman and Lisa Berger explain, "For many years, doctors believed that the expansion and quick contraction of blood vessels in the head were the chief sources of pain. They now know that a lot more is going on, too" with "the trigeminal nervous system and release of brain chemicals such as prostaglandin and serotonin" (195). It would, of course, be more scientifically "objective" to say that heredity and chance make some of us vulnerable to cortical spreading depression, spasms in the vascular system, inflammation, an intense feedback loop of trigeminal nociception, and sensory hyperexcitability, ultimately leaving us with completely senseless but often piercing pain and extreme sensitivity to movement, sound, light, and smells. But I like the poetic precision of expressing how biology feels as if it is complicit with ideology through the portmanteau-term *trigemony* (wouldn't Lewis Carroll approve?). Playing on the name of the troublesome trigeminal nervous system, *trigemony* encompasses the ideologies of silencing pain, as well as the (sometimes literally) paralyzing control of migraine. As if in collusion with the hegemonic forces of educational policies, medical practices, and social prejudice, the attacks subdue the child migraineur.

Trigemony also helps to express an unusual quality of the disorder—it is something so private that no one but the migraineur can perceive it's even happening,[2] except through the efforts of the migraineur to communicate the experience, yet one of the most consistent perceptions communicated is the sense that migraine is an external oppressive force, experienced as if from outside of the body. Perhaps this is a quality of pain in general, merely exacerbated by the lack of external indicators. Elaine Scarry writes that

> the fact that the very word "pain" has its etymological home in "*poena*" or "punishment" reminds us that even the elementary act of naming this most interior of events entails an immediate mental somersault out of the body into the external social circumstances that can be pictured as having caused the hurt.

(1985, 16)

In the past chapter I looked at how some migraineurs have taken up a weapon in this somersault out of the body, how they've been fictionalized and presented to the public through stereotypes and obscuring metaphors. In this chapter I'll look at firsthand expressions of how it feels to be under the oppressive force of migraine, with a particular focus on its consequences for children.

Chronic or severe pain incapacitates other faculties; as Melanie Thernstrom writes, "it kidnaps consciousness, annihilating the ordinary self" (69). Michelle Martinovic, whose attacks began at age five, told me,

> I get annoyed even now when I hear someone say "I think I have a migraine." If you're thinking clearly at all . . . and you're not sure . . . then it's not a migraine. All it takes is one true migraine for you to realize it's a whole different beast.

(personal interview)

Jennette Fulda echoes Nietzsche in her description: "My world was limited to the size of my skull. . . . There was no world outside the headache" (3, 31). Arthur W. Frank says, however, of pain in general,

> Dealing with pain is not war with something outside the body; it is the body coming back to itself. But taking pain entirely into my own body, making it too much my own, carries the danger of becoming isolated in that body.

(2002, 31)

Whether felt as internal or external, the pain of migraine isolates us in the experience.

When the hurt is actually experienced in the head, felt as the seat of our sentience in Western ideology, a kind of existential dilemma occurs. Paula Kamen perfectly captures this paradox in her playfully titled book, *All in My Head: An Epic Quest to Cure an Unrelenting, Totally Unreasonable, and Only Slightly Enlightening Headache* (2005). Throughout the past two centuries, many migraineurs have been presented with the dismissal that "it's all in your head," due to theories of psychosomatic causes and stereotypes about "migraine personality." But Kamen explains that once she understood her migraine condition had become chronic, "something was really wrong. I wanted to believe that the problem was indeed all in my head, but not in my mind" (9). We should not accept that we are victims of pain, but we are not the pain either.

David B. Morris writes, "Chronic pain destroys our normal assumptions about the world. . . . We are helplessly under the control of outside forces" (1991, 71). There are physiological reasons for the sense of migraine pain existing outside of us, out of our heads. Scott Fishman and Lisa Berger explain that the pain of migraine "is not generated in the brain, which has no sensory nerves, but in the nerves of the scalp, face, mouth, and throat, as well as in the blood vessels at the base of the brain" (195). But phenomenologically speaking, we lack the language or even analogy to convey this sense of external oppression. In Gemma Elwin Harris's *Big Questions from Little People and Simple Answers from Great Minds*, a child asks "How does my brain control me?" Neuroscientist Susan Greenfield responds, "'My brain' and 'me' are the same. So one cannot control the other" (102). However, when our will and our body seem to operate at such cross purposes, and our "brain" seems to work against our intentions, we experience the very opposite—an intense sense of identity that is separate from the hell in our heads. The pain is not of our making.

N. Ann Davis writes,

> [I]t is reasonable to suppose that people's inclination to downplay the significance of mental or psychological symptoms stems less from the desire to discount subjective reports and more from views about the will and the nature and extent of individual's control over their thoughts and feelings. Such views attribute great importance, and great power, to individual volition. In its crudest form, this view embodies what I shall call "the myth of the world-transcendent will": the view that what we think or feel is essentially up to us.
>
> (186)

In the abstract, this common response may sound empowering, but to the person wracked with uncontrollable pain, it is downright offensive. Any claim that migraine is "all in our heads" is likely to leave migraineurs, well, hypersensitive about being called hypersensitive.

Nathan Speer explained this split to me as "feeling mad at your body for betraying you," but the migraine "centers you so wholly on it that you can't think of anything else" (personal interview). Marquetta F. Russell described her early experience of migraine, expressing the ambiguity of inner and outer boundaries caused by head pain:

> I had never known terror before. The pain is terrifying . . . I hated that I knew this is what terrorizing pain feels like, where you don't understand what to do, or where it comes from, or how to stop it, or how you can ever get outside of this point. . . . Nothing I had ever felt compared to this. . . . Now I have a different awareness of pain when others are in it – not having any control over what's happening to you . . . and for me it was coming from my body. For other people coming from an outside force.
>
> (personal interview)

One migraineur, Kane Zeller, whom I was able to interview with his mother, Dee Goedert (also a migraineur), recalled that Dee "would bang against the wall to feel the pain on the outside" (personal interview). It's really like being possessed. In fact, Andrew Levy writes that "it's not so much a headache as a possession, my head an occupied territory, and my normal self, a disenfranchised native populace, driven underground" (30). Jennette Fulda describes chronic daily headache as a colonizer crowding out the self: "I was the headache and the headache was me" (12). Ashley Meunchen, the fibers artist whose work I discussed in chapter 1, went as far as saying, "I am a migraine who occasionally gets to be a person" (personal interview). Creating her art exhibit on her migraine experience was an effort in exorcism: "I needed it to be out of me." Such experience frustrates and necessitates imagining boundaries—a barrier protecting the self from that which seems out of one's control.

Trigemony connotes this oppression on a social, phenomenological, and neural level. One needs to feel the ability to push back. Suzanne C. Thompson writes, "[E]xperiments that have separated controllability and predictability have found that controllability has effects over and above the predictability it provides," meaning that we can cope with pain best if we feel as if we have control over it (96). She explains, "[T]he control does not need to be exercised for it to be effective and . . . it does not even need to be real, just perceived, for it to have effects" (89). The strong social control adults have over the conditions in which children experience pain must be corrected to at least enable young persons in pain to have a sense of control. This is especially important in the case of migraine, with which any illusion of control is constantly mocked by the ill-timing of attacks. Far from the popular idea of "having a headache" as an excuse from unpleasant situations, the fact that migraine can be so uncontrollable is especially clear when it prevents us from enjoying the things we love the most—like sunshine, laughter, or punk music.[3] Annecy Crockett, who has had migraine attacks since the age of 6, and who was 10 years old at the time of our second interview, getting attacks every week, shared this relevant page from her diary:

Dear Diary,

Today I woke up in my bed feeling fine. Then out of nowhere a migraine popped into my head. This reminds me of when I got sick right after school got [out] the other day. This particular day was my Christmas party to which I invited my good friends. We all hopped into Mamas car and drove home.

My migraine was getting really bad. I felt that if someone bumped into me I would throw up all over. . . and that's just what I did.

Next, I laid down on the couch sweating all over. I closed my eyes and clenched my teeth forcing back my wails of pain. Soon I fell asleep on our couch waking up to an empty house, I had missed the whole party.

The next day of school wasn't great. The word had gone out to the whole class that I had ruined the party. "And you didn't even invite me," said another girl. My migraines are horrible.

– Annecy

Note that all of the tensions mentioned before are apparent in this diary entry: the child's will is conceptualized as separate and pitted against an intruding pain that has "popped into" her head. Likewise, nine-year-old Christopher described migraine to Elliot Krane: "It's like somebody is inside my head with a boom box" (11). One seven-year-old boy, cited by Leora Kuttner, says it is "like a big monster that is growing like crazy, and there's no room. So it pulls the two sides of his head apart because the monster is getting so big!" (288). Another nine-year-old-boy explained migraine as like "a tyrannosaurus rex bites the head off a brontosaurus. I'm the brontosaurus" (Rovner). Dee Goedert told me that "migraine is violent," which is echoed in three children's descriptions collected by Dorothea Ross and Sheila Ross, analogizing migraine as "like cruel fingers creeping up the back of my neck" at the prodromal stage, "like someone whipping your head" when the pain begins, and "like a sledgehammer is inside your head trying to break out" during full attack (1988, 185).

Children are especially likely to look for visible signs of pain or describe it in highly visualizable terms. Elliot Krane explains that by the time children are five or six years old, "they are fascinated with any visible evidence of pain, such as scars, black and blue marks, scabs, and stitches" (10). Patrick J. McGrath and Kenneth D. Craig found, in their investigation of development affecting pain communication, "the youngest group focused on perceptually dominant physical factors. The slightly older children began to use physical analogies to describe pain" (826). But invisible pain has always demanded explanation, and Esther Cohen identifies the demand as a human tendency for all ages: "The fact that late medieval mystics begged for visible marks of their pain without having physically to inflict it shows an awareness of the power that lay in their bodily sensations," but even more, an awareness of the need for visible proof (212). This example she provides is particularly familiar:

> A sick nun in Ghent suffered such a headache that the back of her head "boiled like a pot on fire" and her eyes, full of fire too, almost popped out of her head. Pain assumed a visible form coming out of the body.
>
> (212)

Visualizing corporeality is expedient in some literary characterizations of headache. Take the example of the tragic figure, Captain Ahab, in *Moby-Dick*. We are supposed to know that his head pain is real because of the scar on his forehead that seems to also discolor his hair—he is marked.[4] Ahab asks the *Pequod*'s blacksmith,

> "[L]ook ye here – here – can ye smoothe out a seam like this, blacksmith," sweeping one hand across his ribbed brow; "if thou coulds't, blacksmith, glad enough would I lay my head upon thy anvil, and feel thy heaviest hammer between my eyes."
>
> (Melville 699)

The violence of his request resembles those reported by migraineurs, but his pain is made palpable, credible by his physical appearance. Likewise, Harry Potter has been diagnosed as a migraineur in a delightfully playful article in the medical journal, *Headache,* by doctors Fred Sheftell et al., who write,

> An attempt by Voldemort to kill Harry as an infant left him with an erythematous frontal scar in the shape of a lightning bolt, which the book cover illustration shows to be just above the medial part of the left orbit.

Unfortunately, this is in the distribution of the first division of the tri-geminal nerve, the locus of several painful headache disorders including migraine.

(2007, 912)

Harry's pain comes from a source of evil outside of his body—Voldemort. In fact, a quick Google search will bring up an image of the card many migraineurs posted on their blogs, which reads, "I have a headache. Voldemort must be close." But the scar is what makes Harry's pain real to the reader and even legitimates his heroism, which Alison Bechdel alludes to in her comic strip "Dykes to Watch Out For" when Mo reads from *Harry Potter* (or "Harry Potty") to a group of youngsters, one of whom asks, "Where's your scar if you're Harry Potter?" (247). She's not trying to pass herself off as Harry, though she does have similar glasses—a coincidence enough to inspire the revealing question about her missing the essential element, his scar (see figure 4.1). When the first film adaptation of *Harry Potter* came out, fans were upset to find the position of the scar changed from the illustrated book cover. Whereas Mary GrandPre's illustrations show Harry's scar on the center of his forehead, it was placed above his left brow in the films at J. K. Rowling's request ("Potter's scar"). That fans would be upset indicates the extent to which that scar is his unique identifier, proof that he can meet with and survive an evil confrontation. And proof that his head pain is real?

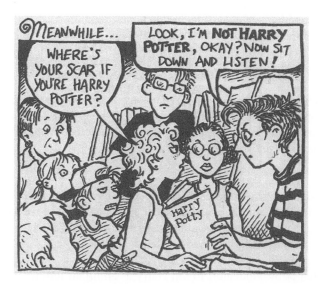

Figure 4.1 From *The Essential Dykes to Watch Out For* by Alison Bechdel. © 2008 by Alison Bechdel. Reprinted by permission of Houghton Mifflin Harcourt Publishing Company. All rights reserved.

Even in works of fiction, where the author might have chosen to take us into the migraineur's mind and describe the suffering, some authors reinforce head pain by outward signs. Andrew Levy writes, "The language of migraine is all outside. What is needed is the language of the inside" (157). The challenge of "seeing" into another's pain is universal, as one pain specialist, Dr. Jason Rowling, told me, "There is no objective evidence" to follow, meaning that there is no certainty about the degree or even the actuality of pain reported by patients—"you just never know" (personal interview). Dr. Joost Haan, a neurologist at Leiden University, told me that in spite of the seemingly deterministic focus of his research in isolating the genetic phenotype for familial hemiplegic migraine, he sees the disorder as a Foucauldian discourse: "as long as migraine doesn't have a test [proof], it will remain *discourse*." More doctors need to actually *see* their patients during an attack, he advises: "[S]eeing a patient during attack was an eye-opener." Even so, he states, "It cannot be measured." According to Dr. Haan, genetic research is meant to "prove that it is migraine." Otherwise, "the only proof exists in words,"[5] in the stories migraineurs tell. Haan says, "The only reason we take it as true is because they are all telling the same story."

Elaine Scarry writes, in "Among School Children," that

> the absence of visible body damage makes it hard for physicians or non-physicians to credit the reality of the patient's pain; the presence of visible body damage may either repel or receive the onlooker's attention, but, in either case, it sits on top of, and obscures, the person in pain.
>
> (23)

Migraineur Caleb Hood explained to me, "You can't show a picture of what's happening in your head—of the inside you can't touch." So it makes perfect sense that images of externalized causes dominate migraine art, including drawings by children, who are more likely than adult migraineurs to be linguistically limited. One of the most common tropes in artwork collected in such books as Podoll and Robinson's *Migraine Art* and Blondin's *Migraine Expressions: A Creative Journey through Life with Migraine* is the nail, hammer, or knife stabbing the eye or forehead. Rather than reflecting migraineurs' exposure to the trope itself, I believe the prevalence of such images indicates an awareness of what is needed to convey the pain to non-migraineurs, which is especially indicative in child migraineurs' diagnostic drawings (Lewis 1996, Stafstrom et al. 2002, 2005, Podoll and Robinson 2008, Wojaczynska-Stanek et al. 2008).

Such images can play an important role in migraine diagnosis, especially for children, as demonstrated by the drawings in figure 4.2, which were made by migraineurs aged 9–12. Stafstrom et al. comment on frame A, where "[a] 9-year-old boy depicts pounding pain inflicted by a hammer and chisel. Note the chiseled appearance of his skull" (2002, 463). Though diagnostic drawings do not necessarily demonstrate degrees of pain, they are pretty clear about the nature of the pounding sensation. They can also express symptoms like phonophobia and photophobia, as in my favorite, E, where a 10-year-old boy depicts "a drum set in

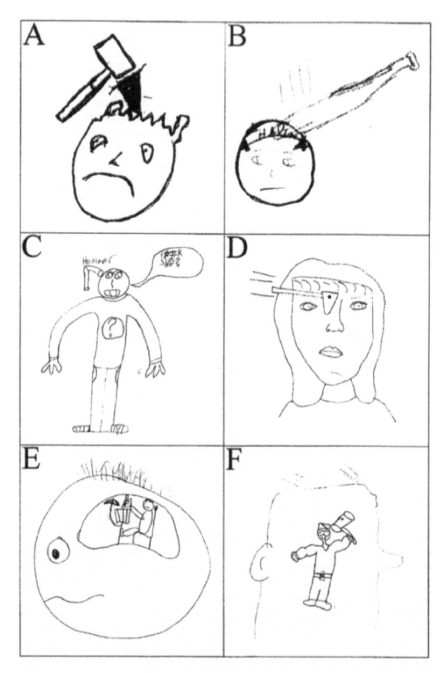

Figure 4.2 Reproduced with permission from *Pediatrics* Vol. 109, page 463 © 2002

my brain" (2002, 463). Diagnostic drawings are also effective at relating visual phenomena of aura. Those who experience prodromal aura might have an entirely unique visual, auditory, tactile, or olfactory hallucination (and sometimes partial blindness or paralysis) every time an attack is coming on; knowing others have this experience, even if it isn't identical in nature, can be comforting.

This need for comfort through community may be one motive for the many posthumous outings of migraineurs in the literature of migraine mentioned in my last chapter, and there has been a tendency toward romanticizing[6] migraine, especially visual aura, in artists as well. Richard Grossinger writes, in *Migraine Auras: When the Visual World Fails*, that "*[m]igraine* is a way of viewing the universe, which may be imposed by a bioneural sequence" (49). Giorgio de Chirico was posthumously "diagnosed" this way (though it is clear that his friends recognized his condition as migraine during his lifetime). His memoirs and paintings radiate with scintillating scotomata, though de Chirico himself "seemed to interpret his [visions] as privileged revelations of another reality" (Podoll 1988, 1672). The visions of Hildegard von Bingen, the medieval mystic, are also explained in a similar diagnostic fashion (Sacks 1992, 53). Grossinger adds that even non-migraining artists have appropriated auratic features in their own aesthetic. Romanticizations of migraine tend to imply migraineurs have greater intelligence and creativity, but Frank Vertosick puts the much-needed practical spin on this tendency:

> The romantic association between migraines and intellectuals at one time had some basis in science. Migraines were once thought to be more common in the mentally gifted, a belief supported by limited epidemiological evidence. This idea has been refuted by more recent studies showing no relationship between migraines and intelligence. . . . To a migraineur, headaches aren't the engines of DeChirico oils, Carroll fables, or beatific visions of the Virgin Mary. They are instruments of torment, nothing more or less.
>
> (21)

Oliver Sacks's book *Migraine* continued and popularized the romanticizing tradition. Punning on an Oliver Sacks title, Tom Shakespeare famously dubbed Sacks "the man who mistook his patients for a literary career" (137). In *Vulnerable Subjects: Ethics and Life Writing*, G. Thomas Couser criticizes Sacks for exploiting his medical subjects for their stories, contributing to their "enfreakment" (79). By exploiting these patients and their stories, Sacks did contribute to making migraine more visible to a general reading public, however. Such stories generate human interest. I find more problematic his seeming erasure of pain by exoticizing individual experiences, especially by selectively focusing on the visual aura[7] of migraineurs (which he, like Charles Dodgson, experienced without the more troublesome symptom of head pain). One example of such erasure through romanticizing is the insistence Sacks makes on recognizing euphoria as a postdromal feature "dramatized by the sense of extreme refreshment, and almost of rebirth, which may follow a severe but compact attack" (31). Surprised by his inclusion of "rebound and refreshment" as a symptom, I asked all of my migraine interviewees whether they had experienced such euphoria. Most were puzzled by the question. None answered in the affirmative. And here's, I think, why: of course they feel refreshed upon waking from a severe attack—this is a rational response to a very basic animal experience: relief from pain. That Sacks hyperdiagnoses such states into his symptomology reveals his own lack of embodied awareness of how extreme pain and its relief naturally affect a person's mood.[8] The inability to comprehend, or resistance to comprehending, the holistic pain experience can lead to romanticizing emphasis on less debilitating auratic features.

Such an impulse might also explain the popularity and problematic receptions of migraine art. In her provocative chapter, "Monsters, Cyborgs, Animals: Crashes, Cuttings, and Migraines," Petra Kuppers admits her discomfort with the diagnostic use of artwork: "Sacks seems to pathologize artistic expressions" (2007, n. 23, 232). And indeed, most of the first avenues for exposure granted artists and audiences presented migraine art as diagnostic fodder. Most problematically, this resulted in artwork appearing unattributed. Klaus Podoll has explained this to me as necessary for protecting the identity of the "patient" not explicitly to devalue the accomplishment of the artist (email, 23 August 2013). Though the context framing such work is regrettably disempowering politically, I would argue that, recontextualized, it is useful to the migraine-viewer. Perhaps this difference in perspective may also hinge on a distinct priority in the politics of invisible disability. Personally, I see migraine art as a refreshingly therapeutic point of connection with others, especially in light of the dearth of accurate or authentic representations. Because such art makes migraine experience more visible, some viewers may be willing to overlook the negatives. If anyone ever made me feel like a freak, it was the teachers, classmates, doctors, and advice-giving strangers who failed to understand or lessen my suffering as a child—not migraine art.

Through art, children can represent phenomena that are very difficult for those of us without aura to understand otherwise. For a unique example, Podoll and Robinson (2008) provide a sample illustration by eight-year-old Hayley Welding depicting two rarer auras—a compressed sense of time (sometimes called "the rushes")[9] and polyopia, wherein the migraineur sees numerous projections of one image (see figure 4.3). Such artwork is not merely diagnostic for doctors or therapeutic to viewers. It can also be therapeutic to the artist, as Helen Neal points out: "[C]hildren find . . . emotional release through drawing and painting. Not only is it a release, but, by expressing their pain graphically, they are given a sense of control over a situation in which they are helpless" (147). Again, the sense of control, even illusory, helps in our struggle against trigemony.

The focus on aura, however, may turn attention away from the problem that migraineurs, with or without aura, agree is the more debilitating factor—the pain. Even Jessica Benzel, the migraineur with the most debilitating prodromal obstacles of anyone I interviewed—"Alice in Wonderland" syndrome, paralysis, and an inability to speak—lists pain just before aura in her answer to my question, "What do you wish non-migraineurs understood better?" responding, "The pain and how debilitating the aura can seem when it's happening" (email). And, in fact, because the auras are more briefly experienced, and more of us have migraine without aura

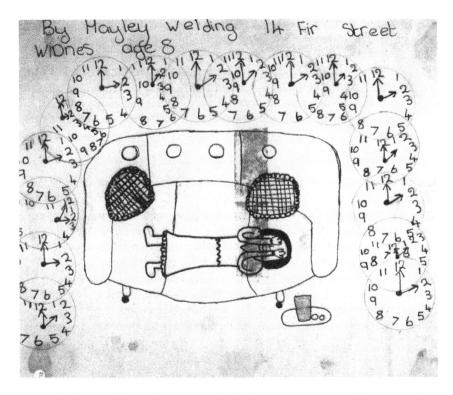

Figure 4.3 Hayley Welding, Migraine Art Collection. Image courtesy of Migraine Action, UK www.migraine.org.uk

(thus the old term "common migraine"), most migraine art seems to focus on the pain; it's just the auras that get sensationalized in writing.

Sensationalizing can enable insensitivity in unexpected ways, like when well-meaning people post comments on migraine websites about how they wish they could experience migraine, or at least aura, for themselves—if only neurological tourism were possible. Such a cringe-worthy moment occurs in the following recollection, which eventually redeems itself in its attention to detail:

Another person, who had heard about scotomata for years, wished he had had one so that he could know what they were like. Then out of the blue he remarked, "Could those bright shapes that crossed my vision in kindergarten have been migraine auras? They left me blinded for a while. I assumed that they were another of those things I wasn't supposed to understand. My teachers were no help on anything else, so I never told them. By George, I guess I had them! I remember the last one was at school around first or second grade. I was amazed no one else talked about this stuff; I figured maybe it was only me."

(Grossinger 55–56)

But for most, the aura is a sign of something much worse coming. In "The Lightning-Rod Man: The Migraine Headache as Heuristic Tool," Paul West's lyrical descriptions of the "cortical movie" he experiences in his "visual cockpit" nevertheless make clear that his lack of control over pain threatens his sense of free will:

> A star of gall in one's head is nothing to be envied, of course, but it has its motley allure, conferring auspices that yield estimable alliances I am not now eager to wish away . . . all of us with migraine headaches, marking time while it marks us.
>
> (294–295, 300)

His lightshow still does not dim his clearer message: "[M]y nuisance is still captain of its fate" (299).

As with power reinforced by consensus, trigemony at times has its corporate collaborators. The pharmaceutical industry is always, sometimes indecipherably, in the shadows, particularly in our age of native advertising. It is so present that Paula Kamen reserves an entire frontispiece for this disclaimer: "NOTE: This book was *NOT* made possible by an unrestricted educational grant from Merck, Allergan, Pfizer, Eli Lilly, Endo Pharmaceuticals, AstraZeneca, Upjohn, Purdue Pharma, OrthoMcNeil, Bayer, Advil, or the icepack industry. Really." But Petra Kuppers makes more serious claims, using migraine art and websites as her example of this often overlooked reality:

> Within this economy of diagnoses and descriptors, advice and medical expertise, migraine art hosted by bodies such as the National Headache Foundation are additions, the human face to word-heavy sites on migraine management (often through drugs). It is interesting how drugs function within this economy of imagery and words. While the creative images seem open as to the origin of migraines, and often focus on social effects and relations caused by the condition, the drug experience traditionally severs these relations. Drug development pinpoints biochemical actions and individual body sites. The Internet itself stands in this double bind. On the one hand, it links wider communities into discourse, and on the other it alienates bodily encounter, replaces actual meetings with virtual ones.
>
> (2007, 147)

The unethical practice of corporately funded medical studies makes getting accurate and helpful information fraught with uncertainty—and though the Internet is a seemingly democratic medium, there is no way for the casual surfer to know how much some information is motivated by pharmaceutical profit.[10] Indeed, unattributed migraine art is an example of a "severed" opportunity for community solidarity. The identity of the artist fades, with his or her name, into the anonymous past as the artwork is "diagnosed" by doctors, not art critics. In fact, some might bristle at the sound of *migraine art* and ague that it fits more in the traditions of outsider art, folk art, and *art brut*. But Kuppers's comments also reveal a complication within disability politics when it comes to discussing pain. Though I agree that the social relations fostered through fellow migraineurs' support should not be severed, I also have never met a migraineur who doesn't want to be "severed" from their pain—no one who actually experiences migraine pain wants to be a member of this club. I challenge you to find one.

A person in pain isn't likely to have the luxury of treating their bodies like a temple and thinking that all drugs are bad, or at least is more likely to think drugs are the lesser evil. Just because pharmaceutical companies are making an unholy profit off our pain, invading our websites, and sometimes the drugs they develop are even worse that what they purport to relieve, that doesn't mean drugs themselves are dispensable for the sake of emancipatory identity and solidarity. This conflict reminds me of one day in a graduate class, where my professor overheard me discussing (with another migraineur) the triptan I'd injected less than an hour before (rather than miss class). She chastised me for two well-meaning, oversimplified, but unfortunately widely believed reasons: first, that drugs merely mask symptoms; second, that those symptoms are indicative of my body telling me to simply change something I'm doing wrong—like how I eat, sleep, or, for example, which classes I should have skipped.[11] But dysfunctional pain is not necessarily telling an experienced and careful migraineur anything but that their cranial vessels and sensory neurons have gone berserk. The causes of migraine are believed, and have been for over a century, to be similar to those of epileptic seizures, yet no one in such a social setting would tell someone with epilepsy to stop masking their symptoms by not taking anticonvulsants. Telling a migraineur that they aren't listening enough to the message of their body's pain is a little like telling someone suffering from phantom limb pain that they should just keep looking for their missing limb.

The very fact that conditions of fluctuating impairment are so changeable is used to blame those affected rather than support social reforms to help the chronically ill better cope and participate fully in school, work, and social life. Joanna Kempner writes that

> almost everyone has well-intentioned, often contradictory, and always illadvised recommendations for those who have serious headache disorders: drink more water, take two aspirin, do yoga, meditate, seek acupuncture and Chinese medicine, alter your diet, take regular exercise, do not exercise strenuously, take vitamins, take herbs, use heat, use ice, use nothing, relax, or, most annoyingly, "just think about something else." Some of these recommendations can help some of the time, but most are useless to the person in serious pain.
>
> (x)

Susan Wendell explains the peril of blaming the sick in her explanation that "unhealthy disabled" persons often have fluctuating impairments:

> Fluctuations in our illnesses and abilities – which can be affected by our emotions, changes in our lives, and stress, but which may occur independently of

them – contribute to the perception that we are responsible for our disabilities. In addition, an abundance of popular theories claim or imply that anyone can control her/his health with the right diet, exercise, attitudes, relationships, or religious beliefs: it follows from most of them that those who are unhealthy are doing something wrong.

(29)

Self-help books are chock-full of this sort of abuse. Take for example, Deb Shapiro's *Your Body Speaks Your Mind*, in which the author bullet-points the top "causes" of migraine as "Fear of failure," "Issues of control and power," "Repression of Feelings," "A fear of participation and involvement," and "A way of getting attention, care, and love" (160–161). This advice was not published in Steinbeck's day for hypothetical women like Bernice Pritchard; it was published in 2006. Jennette Fulda, in her memoir on chronic daily headache, reproduces an excellent range of such offensive advice-giving throughout the book, quipping in response, "I knew the next time someone asked me if they'd discovered what was causing my headache, I was going to reply, 'Other people's advice'" (117).

Well-intended but offensively generalizing advice doesn't just come from those fortunate enough to be blissfully ignorant about uncontrolled pain. Some migraineurs want so badly for what *worked for them* to *work for you* that they forget this frustration in their zealousness. Complicating sincere efforts is the fact that migraine is, as Kempner says, a spectrum disorder:

> Most people who have migraine are on the mild end of the spectrum; they might experience one to three headache days per month and lose some functionality as a result of symptoms. But about a quarter experience severe levels of disability associated with their symptoms.

(5)

This means that some get mild symptoms and misproject their own experience onto those with more severe impairment. Again, well meaning, but the empathy fails. For example, in her otherwise helpful book *Digestive Wellness*, Elizabeth Lipski reports that female migraineurs experience attacks often due to hormonal fluctuation.[12] True, this is why, whereas male migraineurs equal or slightly outnumber females in childhood, in adults only one in four migraineurs is male. But, Lipski dangerously generalizes from her own experience, finding the culprit in birth control pills: "When women stop taking these medications, their migraines typically disappear" (368). Only partly true: hormonal changes only account for some attacks, and certainly not for all migraineurs. Seventy-five percent of females will, in fact, experience a decrease in the incidence of attacks after menopause (not surprisingly, that's the same proportion of female migraineurs who got their first attacks with puberty, not before). But I've come to be wary of anyone who uses *migraines*, *typically*, and *disappear* in the same sentence. This hallmark rhetoric of snake-oil salesmen is unfortunately ubiquitous with the impairment. More to the point of my larger argument, this is of no help to the seven-year-old boy who misses one-third of his school days in a year from attacks.

There is no single remedy or solution that helps all migraineurs—a common lament of patients, parents, and doctors. And for child migraineurs developing a coping strategy can be frustrated by ambiguities in diagnosis and resulting delays in any treatment plan. Charles Barlow writes that even with early "onset of symptoms from 4 months through the 2nd year," seeking medical help is delayed: "In most instances, the child was first seen from 1 to 10 years after onset" (92). This is partly because children with migraine can have briefer attacks, the pain is sometimes less clearly unilateral, and "[m]ost children had no prodromal symptoms" (Aromaa 1998, 1731). But Barlow also indicates that

> [t]he diagnosis of juvenile migraine is purely clinical and rests upon the history, which in turn relies primarily upon the patient's observations and memory and upon the determination and attitude of the physician. . . . [I]t represents the most serious weakness of . . . studies of migraine in general.
>
> (94)

That an understanding of the impairment requires an individual history means that children might have to suffer longer in order to articulate and discover why they are suffering (a common problem with chronic illnesses). Christopher Eccleston and Peter Malleson add that particularly in the cases of children, doctors first need to factor out life-threatening causes, thus delaying and sometimes adding to the sense that patients are getting the run-around: "Doctors concerned about missing a serious underlying disease invest time and energy in investigating the child and referring to specialists for their evaluation. During the time spent in this 'diagnostic vacuum,' the child often receives little appropriate pain management" (1408). Fears of masking symptoms may keep children in pain, increasingly the likelihood of developing further pain complications later on.

Although diagnosis is often seen in disability politics as a trap that medicalizes identity, it is often a welcome relief to those who have endured without help for too long. One mother of a 16-year-old with abdominal migraine told Elliot Krane, "No one wants their child to be sick, but I just wanted the doctors to put a name to what was going on" (37). Jean Jackson writes, "Because pain is invisible and unmeasurable, some of the patients whose cases were not crystal clear asserted that they would have preferred having a known problem, even a serious one" (340). One chronic pain patient, Sandra Glynn, tells Jackson she was delighted to finally hear a doctor tell her, "Sandra, you absolutely have a problem." Jackson explains, "Cancer was preferable, I was told more than once, because it is a known danger with treatment possibilities" (340). Such confessions speak to the desperation of patients with chronic and invisible conditions that thwart efforts to cope, compacting the danger of simply accepting a diagnosis if the resulting treatment doesn't help or is unnecessarily invasive. Donald J. Lollar and Rune J. Simeonsson warn to still approach a received diagnosis as a working strategy not a determination: "[A]ssigning a diagnosis may reveal little about the functional characteristics of a child or adolescent. Diagnoses are associated with symptomology, often unrelated to function" (323). And, particularly in the now highly specialized field of neurology, there has been a tendency to prescribe experimentally, off-label, rather than to focus on comprehensive, creative options for alternatively assisting young migraineurs in gaining control over their condition.

Subtler levels of denial complicate the process as well. Parents of children with disabilities report that doctors are likely to "discount" and "dismiss" their concerns, especially when about "infants and young children" (Green 2015). Sometimes parents can complicate the process of treating a child's chronic or invisible impairment:

> Fear and frustration are often fueled by unhelpful or inaccurate diagnoses such as "functional" or "psychosomatic" pain. Families often interpret these labels as blaming them for the child's pain, and the labels tend to reinforce their need to move from doctor to doctor in search of a different diagnosis or cure. The path to chronicity of pain is characterized by failed attempts to adjust and cope with uncontrollable, frightening, and adverse experience. Over time it is the weight of this experience that leads the patient to develop concomitant symptoms of chronic pain, physical disability, anxiety, sleep disturbance, school absence, and social withdrawal.
>
> (Eccleston 1408–1409)

Negative consequences of early prolonged helplessness in a diagnostic vacuum merit serious consideration for ensuring lifespan health.

One of the most consistent explanations for the difficulty of diagnosing child migraine is the assumption that it is not as severe as adult migraine. Even Bille makes this claim (28). This may be true in general, though I'm not sure how, either way, this could be measured or empirically proven. All I can say to this claim is that I've experienced severe migraine as a child and as an adult, and the fact that I now have the power to advocate for myself medically has given me a profound sense of how much worse it was to be a child with migraine. For me there is no comparison. Invisibly suffering through severe migraine without relief, in a culture that cannot even recognize its own collusion with trigemony, is something I'm glad I'll never have to personally endure again—but there are children doing just that every day. The consequences of ableism, ageism, marginalization, and pain are just as urgent now as ever.

Pain has proven a difficult and fascinating subject politically. We've already seen how both pain and anesthesia have historically been used to control children in chapter 2, and Martin Pernick identified predictions of twentieth-century control through medications from the nineteenth-century model he studied: "Many nineteenth-century asylums reported using anesthetics to control patients. . . . Although ether and chloroform never became as important a means of institutional control as tranquilizers are today" (229). Whereas Martin Pernick dubbed the nineteenth century "the Age of Pain," Ivan Illich famously depicted the twentieth century as a period of numbed passivity in a culture obsessed with "minimizing pain" (151). Michael Taussig nuanced this sort of logic:

> It is not, as Illich maintains, for example, that patients lose their autonomy. Far from it. Instead, what happens is that the modern clinical situation engenders a contradictory situation in which the patient swings like a pendulum between alienated passivity and alienated self-assertion.

(9)

This pendulum swing of agency is particularly complicated when the person in need of safe medical treatment is a minor. Getting appropriate pain management in the United States in the twenty-first century requires enlightened medical consumerism and advocacy for the young, which means that adults have to recognize child pain *as pain.*

Pain, being invisible, is not only easy to selectively ignore but often projected onto supposed sufferers we would rather put "out of their pain," that is, out of sight. Perhaps this is one reason the case of Bob Flanagan is so often referenced in disability studies. This "supersadomasochistic" performance artist with cystic fibrosis forced his audience to witness his performative pain, modeling a liberatory response to illness. Though masochism is not a practical option for most of us, Flanagan modeled the power of a coping strategy that many can identify with. But there's one thing critics tend to overlook when they review his documentary, *Sick: The Life and Death of Bob Flanagan, Supermasochist* (1997): he admits that the pain he enjoys, like his sexplay, is consensual—by his own admission, he's not really out of control. What makes watching him die so unspeakably wrenching is that in the end he can no longer control, enjoy, or even tolerate, his pain—there is no safe word that will stop it. As the pendulum of control swings, Bob Flanagan, triumphant supermasochist, was also a subject embodied with disease, and not someone who chose to uncritically embrace it or all pain (he had excruciating headaches from lack of oxygen). Exactly two months before his death he wrote, "I'm sick of being Mr. Good Patient. Gimme drugs" (Flanagan 154). And his final sentence in *The Pain Diary* is "I'm going for a late night dip in Dilaudid" (173). What I admire about Bob Flanagan is not just his humorous ability to provoke much-needed critical insight, but his bold and unpretentious honesty. His shock effect frustrates any effort to fit him to his former "poster boy" image or even contemporary efforts in disability studies to celebrate resilience as rejection of allopathic therapy. Robert McRuer writes that Flanagan's poem "Why" (powerfully performed in the documentary) "remains a slap in the face to any classic disability overcoming narrative" (186). Flanagan proves that pain requires performing a different sort of agency than that employed by what Susan Wendell calls the "healthy disabled" who understandably resist the medicalization of their healthy bodies. In contrast, "some very much want to have their bodies cured, not as a substitute for curing ableism, but in addition to it" (18). Although I'm uncomfortable placing migraineurs in the category of "unhealthy disabled," as the "illness" is a fluctuating reality, I haven't yet met a migraineur who would pass up a cure, and I certainly don't fault their politics for it.

I also don't see the person in pain who grasps for control a dupe of allopathic medicine. Petra Kuppers asks, "If pain does indeed concretize the body, foreground it experientially, why should this be seen as an immobilizing prison to trap the subject in?" (2007, 86). Bob Flanagan dramatized how persons living with pain can at least control how they react to it, setting an important, positive example. In fact, some contemporary pain clinics use such skills to foster the agency of their patients:

> They are now more able to cope with the pain than they had been because they have come to see such coping as within their power: "Pain" controlled me, now I control my pain. . . . [T]hey say they cannot make the pain go away, but they can control the circumstances of the pain experience to a certain extent.
> (Jackson 1992, 158)

Children dealing with intractable pain (and those they depend upon for help) need to know this: "It all boils down to giving children some control over or some say in the painful situation" (Krane 14). And this is quite possible. Studies indicate that by age six children are reliable administers of medication when given control: "[L]etting kids administer their own opioids does *not* increase drug complications. . . . It's anxious parents who actually mess things up. They tend to either over- or underdose their children unless they receive a rigorous education program first" (Foreman 85). Just caring is not enough in the struggle to help a child in pain.

Pain might not be a prison, but it frustrates our efforts to be ourselves or even resist drugs we might think are bad for us, which can be confusing with a condition like migraine, which, as one neurologist was fond of telling me, "won't kill you." (She was either lying or not in the loop: though uncommon, some migraineurs die from complications from early migraine drugs, others, usually young-adult migraineurs, from even rarer migraine-induced stroke.[13]) When quality of life is so threatened a person in pain may comprehend different stakes and be more willing to make what seem to be necessary compromises. Pain relief is, in some cases, an offer you can't refuse. David B. Morris observed at a pain clinic that "[p]ain seemed capable of dissolving otherwise rock-hard resistances. I never saw anyone refuse to sign the consent form. Patients did not flinch at hypodermic needles so long and thick that (even from across the room) they resembled hollow barbeque skewers" (1991, 68). Sometimes one simply has to cave.

Of course pain is political, but we are not just political beings. Shaun Best writes that

> even within an emancipatory politics of disability, people have bodies and our bodies are often fragile and feel pain. . . . Not all medical intervention is patronizing or demeaning. To recognize the existence of biologically based realities is not to accept biological dysfunction as the sole cause of disability.
> (170)

Michael Taussig puts it this way: "My disease is a social relation, and therapy has to address that synthesis of moral, social, and physical presentation" (4). What makes migraine an invisible "disability" is the inability of anyone to make migraine simply "disappear," the unwillingness of our culture to make concessions toward conditions necessary for our alternative ability, but also oppressive silencing through age-, gender-, race-, and class-coded inequities and expectations for stoicism in the face of prolonged pain.

Social denial of pain is just another side of wanting to see others "out of their pain." Elaine Scarry explains that "the obscenity of the hurt may drown out our apprehension of the nonobscenity of the person beyond" (2006, 15). When the person in pain is a child, the general public seems even less capable of responding appropriately. In her comparison of magazine advertisements for medical professionals with those for a popular audience, Scarry notes, "The idea of a child in pain is perhaps to medical advertisers what the idea of any person in pain is to commercial advertisers: it appears to inhibit the otherwise habitual reflexes," but "commercial advertisements using children are often among the least believable" (1994, 37–39). As one example, she reprints a medical ad for a painkiller that consists of a simple headshot of a young girl with an adorable smile, gesturing as if to signify she is carefree. Scarry responds, "That this person should have had pain seems intolerable; that she did have pain is something the viewer does not even wonder about; that she is free of it now is self-evident. How could we disbelieve her?"(1994, 38). And, of course, the reason we see a painfree child in an advertisement for pain medications is not just because it gives us hope of helping others like her to control their pain; it is also because we do not want to see a child in pain. The general public, unfortunately, likes to see "poster children," not children in pain. So, often, they simply don't see children in pain.

Tobin Siebers has written that "[t]he fear of pain is often the beginning of oppression. But pain can also be the beginning of compassion. The idea is not to dismiss compassion as if it were oppression but to think about the difference between them" (2010, 190). As adults we must override our fears in order to counter oppression, and we must educate ourselves to be more compassionate. Michael Taussig writes, "As it oscillates between being my property and my being, especially when diseased, my body asks me questions which the physicians never ask or answer: 'Why me?' 'Why now?'" (4). Children ask these questions, too, but I think the unsatisfying answers one can intuit must be far more difficult for children to accept. Elliot Krane explains, "Preschoolers also think that their parents, grandparents, and other authority figures know exactly what hurts and how much, and that they can automatically fix it" (10). How much more frightening and alienating, then, is the uncontrolled pain of migraine to a child who cannot understand why such supposedly all-powerful care is being withheld? This unanswered question, and recognizing that in fact adults are powerless to help, can be equally terrifying.

The uncertainty of diagnosis, help, or even having their impairment affirmed by a believing adult can be devastating to children with untreated migraine. A case in point is that of Matthew, whose migraine "presented before the age of 2 years" (Slap-Shelton 355). He was not diagnosed until he was eight years old, initially misdiagnosed with "pervasive developmental disorder" (356). In her analysis of Matthew's case, Laura Slap-Shelton writes that he "was described as a child whose internal pressure for perfection increased with stress;" episodes occurred during "periods of high stress," complicated by learning difficulties such as "weak delayed verbal memory" (356, 359). Ultimately she concludes that as a result of prolonged exposure to untreated migraine, the abdominal symptoms became particularly exacerbated in a "phobia of eating, which became associated with pain. His controlling and demanding behaviors were also understood as deriving from a need for internal control in reaction to his many years of uncontrolled and unpredictable pain" (356). Some delays in diagnosing children with migraine harken back to the stubborn persistence of mind-body dualism. Abdominal symptoms are more likely to dominate in children's experience, leading to what for some is a separate diagnosis or "migraine equivalent," called "abdominal migraine." In her *Gut Feminism*, Elizabeth Wilson uses childhood abdominal migraine as a model of how symptoms get rhetorically repackaged in shifting contexts: "[A] condition ordinarily known to be in the head has found its way to the gut. Overseer and underbelly are already confused. . . . Which is to say, the periphery is interior to the center; the stomach is intrinsic to mind" (13–14). No wonder Ashley Meunchen couldn't tell me how young she was when she started having attacks. She was not diagnosed until she was 10 years old. Until then, like others I've spoken with, she "didn't have the word for it." Children often linger in this diagnostic vacuum. I, for one, recall doctors saying they "couldn't be sure" as I never had an attack during an EEG. But my symptoms were those of a common migraine (not just abdominal)—no different from my grown-up version. It baffles me now to think of why they even felt an EEG was necessary for such a common and distinctive combination of symptoms other than my young age presenting them with an unnecessary obstacle. I believe, like Elizabeth Wilson, that "[a]bdominal migraine is no more a variant of classical cerebral migraine than classical migraine is a deviation from abdominal pain" (15). Migraine is an integrated, whole-body experience with individual derivations—a spectrum disorder that many adults are simply disinclined to recognize in children.

Complicating trigemony is the fact that so many "authority figures" refuse to even acknowledge that child migraine even exists. All but two of the migraineurs I interviewed (significantly the son of a nurse and the daughter of a neurologist) heard repeated and staunch dismissals like "children don't get migraines" from a teacher, relative, or even parent during their childhood. Dorothea M. Ross and Sheila A. Ross found in their analysis that parents "actively discouraged the discussion of pain events," leading to undiagnosed migraine (182). They reason, "This apparent inaccuracy may reflect a reluctance on the part of the parents and pediatricians to have the term *migraine* in the child's records" (185). But the abuse they suffer often goes deeper than denial; sometimes adults, whether out of helplessness or indifference, get angry at the child who tries to reeducate their assumptions of all pain being functional or kids not suffering from invisible pain. One day, when Kane Zeller was in the fourth grade, parents were invited to the school and the teacher asked her students to stand up individually and tell them what they'd been learning in class. When it was his turn, Kane stood and said, "Trying to survive the day with a migraine." The teacher was visibly angry. Kane's mother whispered an explanation to me: "[T]heir answers were supposed to be positive" (Goedert). What Kane's teacher didn't understand is that Kane's statement *was* positive.

When Annecy Crockett, who began getting migraine attacks at age six, was eight years old, she also experienced the wrath of disbelieving authority after she missed too much school. I asked her how the school nurse responded, and she said the "nurse only deals with Band-Aids and cuts," and usually wasn't at the school anyway (in our small town they rotate schools, so there's often not one on call), but her teacher and principal took the situation into their own hands in punitive fashion. Annecy reports,

> They took me in this room and said "Hey, we know that you've been lying because you've been sick too many times. We know that you just want to stay home for fun." But I had no idea what they were talking about. I said, "I'm really sick." Then they said "we'll send the cops to your house – we don't care, you just need to tell us that you're faking." But I didn't because I wasn't.
> (personal interview, 2 January 2013)

This is coercive interrogation at worst and at best slanderous indifference. When Annecy showed these adults the hospital band still on her wrist from the MRI she missed school for, they claimed that even it was fake. After this, Annecy left to attend a different school, where she doesn't "want the same thing to happen." Now she has fewer sick days, but that is partly because she's "less likely to say something" if she is sick (2013). This is how trigemony entraps.

Andrew D. Hershey identifies some of the biggest problems for child migraineurs in U.S. schools during our authoritarian era, including "Zero tolerance restrictions (cannot have the medications with them)," "Absent or limited access to school nurse," and "Teachers doubting headache" (2010, 260). I want to stress how destructive such a setting is for students with invisible disabilities; and these conditions are practically designed to create the perfect nerve storm in child migraineurs. In a 1992 survey of school nurses about their treatment of child headache at school, Francis J. DiMario found that "[a]nalgesic was administered routinely only by 10%, and about a quarter of respondents felt 'constrained by school policy'" in such cases, "wanting more latitude" (279, 281). At least "31% routinely allowed the child to rest or sleep," which, from reports I've heard, has gotten worse in the decades since the study. These numbers speak to an abysmal lack of understanding about childhood headache and the ways in which administrators might not even recognize that such policies are woefully insufficient for dealing with child pain and invisible disability. Gaye Tuchman argues, "[T]oo often teachers scapegoat children with invisible differences and so decrease an outcast's ability to fit in" (Tuchman 11). Even the most sensitive teachers can unknowingly pass their own stress and prejudices to the students, resulting in discrimination and adding to the complications of their impairments (or at least, impaired students and their classmates are very likely to feel the difference perceived by their teachers).

For many child migraineurs one solution is to change schools, as Annecy did: "[N]ot infrequently children become free from symptoms when they change their teacher or their class or leave the school" (Bille 1967, 24). When my own migraine attacks became debilitating in fourth grade, I was lucky to be able to enroll instead in an alternative school, where there were no grades (letter grades or grade levels—all classrooms were fourth, fifth, and sixth graders combined); in fact the only kind of assessment that existed at my new elementary in the mid-1970s was self-assessment: we made individualized weekly contracts with the teacher for our work and checked the "answers" ourselves or with our peers. My migraines became much less frequent, and I was even able to participate in activities again. But unfortunately most children, especially today, do not have these options. They should. For a young migraineur to be held to punitive attendance quotas and not have nursing staff available, or even a quiet room in which to rest, is bad enough, but educating teachers who are so misinformed about child migraine as to be abusive should be an easier-to-attain and high-priority goal—there's simply no excuse for "doubting headache."

To an onlooker, the child suffering through a migraine attack might seem well behaved if a little withdrawn, and teachers may appreciate her stillness and quiet rather than recognizing in that behavior an avoidance of sound or movement, which cause more pain. When this child has endured enough and asks for help, adults must be capable of recognizing the validity of self-report. Studies indicate that, far from being liars and fakers about "sick days," children are reliable at describing symptoms: "Children themselves are good reporters of their complaints, if they are only given the opportunity and time to report" (Aromaa 1735). Carolyn S. Crow also found that "children's pain perspectives could be developmentally ordered, coded, and scored reliably, and with validity" (33). Anne Gaffney and Elizabeth A. Dunne report that their study found "children do not merely repeat their parents' health-related sayings . . . [C]hildren's self-reported views on pain would seem to be . . . valid" (106). Joanna Bourke argues that even when lacking a ready vocabulary for expressing pain, children "were found to possess extremely rich figurative pain-languages" (2014, 153). It's sad that targeted studies are even necessary to indicate that we should listen to children and respect their input on their healing needs. Gary Walco et al. advise that when in doubt, we should defer to the child: "Adults are often considered more reliable in reporting children's pain than are children. The concern may be that children may feign or exaggerate suffering to obtain some secondary gain," but "[i]f there are discrepancies between a child's report of pain and the observation of a parent or physician, it is best to defer to the child's perspective" (1994, 541–542). If one is aware of the risks of untreated pain, perhaps the stakes will be high enough to err on the side of trust.

Pain behavior is extremely complicated—only exacerbated and developed further by the questioning and distrust adults default to so easily when dealing with children. When children internalize this lack of trust they may indeed use pain behavior to regain control they perceive is lost. Helen Neal describes this commonly recognized assumption: "Children quite early learn how to manipulate indifferent parents through pain" (87). We've all heard the not-so-authentic wails of a protesting child, and probably even recall playing sick ourselves once or twice as a kid. Invisible pain complicates this precarious boundary of trust, Lonnie K. Zeltzer explains, when there is no apparent physical cause or disease found: "[Y]ou were forced to conclude that the child was just faking it to get attention or that there was an underlying psychological cause. . . . Even today, many physicians still use this outdated model to diagnose pain" (2005, 5). Chronic pain patients of all ages experience this distrust:

> Most patients are all too aware of possible suspicion on the part of others that they may be making more of their pain problem than they need to. . . . Many also say they are demoralized by their unending pain and their many memories of people hinting or saying outright that their problem is not one of "real" pain from a "real" cause, or at least not entirely.
>
> (Jackson 1992, 147)

In children this can lead to distrusting adult motives and power, a less acknowledged cause of acting out. Michael Nutkiewicz found that "[t]he oral testimony responses of pediatric chronic pain patients show that children believe physicians are unable or unwilling to recognize the experiential dimensions of pain" (20). These issues are often built up during a childhood of pain, and yet so many adults forget, when speaking with children in pain, that their word may be all they have to go on.

Trigemony implies both the seeming inevitability of intractable migraine and social factors, like the misprojected suspicion of "faking," that collude with it by ignoring and not adapting to the basic needs (and human rights) of child migraineurs, exacerbating pain and further isolating the child. Environmental triggers reflect a culture in which child migraineurs must adapt instead, often by enduring protracted or severe untreated pain. I was surprised at how largely fears of a next attack dominated the emotions of the migraineurs I interviewed. Studies support that migraine is "comorbid" with, and some say actually causes, a host of other lifelong problems: post-traumatic disorders (Haas and Sovner 1969), "crippling" fear (Blau 1984), depression and panic disorder (Langeveld[14] 1996). Migraine is also associated with environmental factors, such as head trauma (Haas and Sovner 1969), bullying (Metsähonkala 1998), and emotional abuse (Tietjen et al. 2010). In three of the cases from my interviews, the subjects began getting attacks after head trauma. One example encompasses many of these socially avoidable causes.

Leon Frederick was nine years old one summer when another kid above him on a playground piece said, "Hey fat-ass, dodge this" and dropped a cinder block on Leon's head: "It was a bloody mess. My whole T-shirt was just blood" (personal interview). Leon needed 10–15 staples to close the wound. The bully who shoved the block was not punished. When school started so did frequent migraine attacks, which lasted "a few days at a time." In spite of the severity of his attacks, and the fact that he had an aunt with migraine, half of his family "was in complete denial of it." Frederick says that his grandmother would insist that "children can't get migraines—you're just faking it." When he'd vomit his father would ask, "Why'd you do that?" as if he had some control or had willed it. Suspicion from those he most depended upon had a lasting effect: "It made me lose some of the trust that I had because many adults discounted what I was trying to tell them. I would say that is one of the biggest troubles I had when I was younger. When you lose the people you trust, your worldview changes completely" (email). The belief that children don't get migraines or that they aren't a debilitating experience only alienates them more. Leon has been a migraineur ever since. His case hints to how interconnected our school experiences, social surroundings, and the need for emotional support are in cases of childhood migraine. Heredity is a strong factor, but environment can heap on triggers. How badly and how often migraine afflicts us is something our culture has a responsibility to diminish. Rather than growing up with a chronic illness in an empathetic community that teaches interdependence through trust, trigemony unfortunately taught Leon instead that "showing any sign of pain was weakness."

The wimp factor

An often unspoken but harsh reality is that if it weren't for industrial development and the rise of child protectionism, those with difficult births, precarious infancies, and early chronic illness would be in even worse shape. Histories and folklore are filled with evidence that children born with "birth defects," "disability," and inexplicable "failure to thrive" have been vulnerable to abandonment and infanticide (Boswell 1988, Eberly 1991). In fact, Joyce Underwood Munro argues that changeling lore may have evolved as a narrative justification for such practices:

> [T]he changeling is a traditional model of the child who fails to thrive. The changeling embodies the idea of the failure of the parent-infant bond and the physical consequences that flow from that failure. By embodying what is not seen, that unknown which is therefore invisible, the changeling renders it visible.
>
> (252)

Though made more socially palatable in fairy stories, "changelings" were thought by parents to be "ill" spawn who had been swapped with their own healthy offspring by a devil or goblins, the solution for which was to abandon them or "change" them back with fatal doses of homeopathic remedies. The fact that supposed "healthy" infants didn't return (but the actual ill one died in the process) seems to be left unaddressed in many versions, belying that the primary problem was considered resolved.

Anthropologist and primatologist Sarah Blaffer Hrdy considers the fate of such offspring within the larger context of animal behaviors:

> Many mammalian mothers can be surprisingly selective about which babies they care for. A mother mouse or prairie dog may cull her litter, shoving aside a runt; a lioness whose cubs are too weak to walk may abandon the entire litter.
>
> (70)

Hrdy explicitly includes humans in this observation. In fact, she argues that humans stand out amongst the Great Apes as unique in the practice of abandonment and infanticide:

> Although human infants are born with the same grasping reflex that other apes have, they lose it shortly after birth. Furthermore, unlike any other ape, a mother in a hunter-gatherer society examines her baby right after birth and, depending on its specific attributes and her own social circumstances (especially how much social support she is likely to have), makes a conscious decision to either keep the baby or let it die.
>
> (72)

Richard Dawkins reduces this life-or-death moment to a blunt cost-benefit analysis, also applying the term "runt" to human cases (125–126). I use the term to press for awareness that children who are granted the investment of parental care might glean on some level their unique indebtedness in the colder light of unspoken calculations surrounding the extra early dependency that results from some impairments or special medical needs. One migraineur I interviewed, Jan Isenker, who has extreme dietary sensitivities and multiple chronic conditions requiring specialized care, recalls at a young age offering her prized silver dollar collection to her parents in order to help defray the cost of medical bills: "I felt bad about the money . . . I was special needsy already . . . I think I kind of just sucked it up" (personal interview). It was a painful memory to her, not because of the ineffectual gesture, but because she could recall how deeply she had sensed herself as a burden.

Frank T. Vertosick imagines a place for child migraineurs within natural histories and even bleaker prehistories:

> While evolutionary pressures don't matter for degenerative illnesses that limit the survival of the elderly, they would certainly come to bear on a common debilitating condition affecting the very young. Lying helpless with a devastating headache for many hours couldn't have been safe behavior for primitive humans. Migraineurs would have been more prone to being devoured by wild beasts. Or spurned by their societies as non-productive malingerers.
>
> (27)

Fighting against assumptions that we are weak or sickly runts takes up a lot of a child migraineur's energy. These impressions are often unspoken but absorbed through our culture, in which one being so debilitated by senseless pain is often viewed as "weak, lazy, or crazy" (Jackson 1992, 160) or "childish, self-indulgent, and weak" (Jackson 2005, 340). And there could be a slight truth to the idea that child migraineurs have a thing or two in common with runts in the nonhuman animal world. Minna Aromma reports that "Silanpää and coworkers [(1983)] found that smallness for gestational age was predictive of headache occurring at preschool age" (27), and Bral adds, "Often, [child migraineurs] are born either prematurely or after a complicated pregnancy" (37). John Boswell reports that during the Middle Ages, "a difficult birth" was enough to motivate oblation, the practice of abandoning infants to monasteries (299).

However, far from being "cry-babies" and "bellyachers," so-called runts can be quite tough. Though the teacher might see a child migraineur as a student who keeps coming to them complaining of a simple headache, the migraining student is more than likely passing as long as he can, only asking for help once it is impossible to maintain composure sitting in a noisy classroom. This over-sight is complicated by the decreased tolerance for restlessness in children we see in American classrooms today, where a quiet, suffering child is off the radar of an overwhelmed teacher prejudiced by the ideal of controllable childhood; Toby Miller writes that "diagnosis pathologizes children who were previously viewed as normal or mischievous. . . . Today's fuzzy boundaries differentiating the feisty child from the ill one are viewed as problematic" (145). Children also learn at a young age to be stoic—that others won't tolerate whining: "The notion that physi-cians prefer 'stoic' pain description is supported by a study first completed at the Massachusetts Eye and Ear Infirmary in 1966 and followed up in 1974. In that study, patients who reported symptoms stoically were assumed to need medical help more urgently than patients who described more symptoms, acknowledged illness and complained of pain" (Lack 56). Trigemony trains even the youngest patients to be tough.

Michael John Coleman, founder of M.A.G.N.U.M., the National Migraine Association, began getting attacks at age six. He writes of the pressures to main-tain once he was a veteran migraineur in high school:

> That sick feeling in my gut wanted to make me vomit, but not in front of my classmates. The pounding would start, like being hit by a baseball bat every thirty or forty seconds. It was amazing that I passed my classes! The pain would get so bad that I would grab a clump of my hair and pull as hard as I could to distract myself from the pain. I felt like I was going to rip a patch of scalp from my head. . . . I would suffer wave after wave of nausea, and I felt like if I could just vomit, I would feel so much better. But never in the classroom in front of the healthy kids, no never that. Never that, because sick people are weak in the eyes of a high school child, and weakness makes you a target of abuse.
>
> (Roberts 45)

In spite of the hardship of the attack itself, much of the challenge depicted by Cole-man is trying to pass as "healthy" for as long as he can. The internalized awareness of "weakness" and fear of being labeled "sick" is one of the more complicated and generally unvoiced problems child migraineurs face. Child culture is tense with unspoken bias against perceived weakness and smallness.

Classmates can be just as insensitive toward child migraineurs as adults who fail to help. This is especially true for boys: "Stress in school was most strongly associ-ated with migraine in girls, and peer relationships were most strongly associated with migraine in boys" (Metsähonkala 225). The peer relationships that trigger attacks are commonly bullying exchanges: "Children with migraine and children with nonmigrainous headache both reported more often being bullied in school, stress in school, and problems in getting along with other children than children without headache" (222). This is not to say that girls don't bully: in fact, Annecy Crockett told me that "mean is the new nice" at her school, where classmates think her headaches make her "superweird." The pack can turn on those categorized as runts quite quickly and with lasting effects.

While adult culture has upheld the ideal of a silent and controllable child, child subcultures can ritualize abusing those perceived as "runts." In the 1960s, Peter and Iona Opie collected and published British children's "exerting games," including "tussles."[15] One example of particular relevance is the following description of a play-battle on some school steps:

> The attackers grab them by their legs and pull them down, sit on them, and pulverise them. Then the other gang comes down from the steps, and strives to rescue their friends, while my friend and I nip round the back and claim the steps. "Come on you miserable runts," we say, and one of the runts runs up the steps, only to be thrown over the side of the railing. By then the others from our gang are with us, dragging one or two hostages by the hair. These we rough up a bit.
>
> (234)

A thirteen-year old further explains the importance of taking a beating: "If you are lucky to get away without any affliction then your gang bashes you up because you have not fought well" (234). The Opies argue that such games demonstrate "the pride that the young take in the practice of stoicism" and enduring pain (233). It is no wonder then that around the same time, one psychoanalyst would generalize that "inhibited rage is almost always associated with headache symptoms" (Adams 1967, 139).

It is not just within public child cultures and schoolrooms that children are made to feel outcast and assigned runtly roles within groups. Justin Torres extends the analogy of domestic violence in this intimate way when he describes his own alienation and mistreatment within his "litter" in *We the Animals* (2011). When he and his brothers watch a litter of kittens, his older brother asks, "How long before they jump the runt?" (107). Torres explains the terror and estrangement that results:

> They both sniggered, and they were sniggering at me, the fay, the runt of the litter; we were once those kittens – three thick, three warm. And we bloodfought over a tin can of pet milk. And jump the runt was a trick as mean as any they pulled on me.
>
> (107)

Subtle outcasting to abuse within the family is often unspoken and so suppressed that the internalized curse results in rage over time. Alice Miller writes of

Nietzsche's childhood migraines as inspiring his later work through suppressed rage:

> [A] protracted cry for liberation from lies, exploitation, hypocrisy. . . . No one – least of all Nietzsche himself – could see how he had suffered from all this as a small child. But his body labored unremittingly under this burden. No one could have realized that the actual source of his suffering was the mendacious morality that governed his everyday life.
>
> (2006, 47)

R. F. de Almeida and P. A. Kowacs write that Anne Frank, whose attacks, like Nietzsche's, are documented as beginning at age 13, was "a child who had fragile health," and they diagnose her "disabling pains" as migraine (1216). Looking at her diary, it is clear her migraine attacks followed her menstrual cycle, but her entries suggest aggravating environmental and resulting emotional factors:

> I'm boiling with rage, and yet I musn't show it, I'd like to stamp my feet, scream, give Mummy a good shaking, cry, and I don't know what else, because of the horrible words, mocking looks, and accusations which are leveled at me every day, and find their mark, like shafts from a tightly strung bow, and which are just as hard to draw from my body . . . Leave me in peace, let me sleep one night at least without my pillow being wet with tears, my eyes burning and my head pounding.
>
> (30 January 1943, 353)

Anne Frank's case indicates how complicating both the conflict of her life experience (everyday threat of trauma and uncertainty) as well as the more mundane and common conflicts within families can be in creating unresolved tensions and rage affecting migraine. But rather than being recognized as indicators of family and socio-structural problems, such expressions are often clinically neutralized in discourse. Nietzsche's biographer credits him with "migraine-enduring fortitude" (26), and certainly no one would call Anne Frank a whiner, but even expressed rage is silenced in psychotherapeutic readings. In 2006 Richard Grossinger would write, "Suppressed rage and fake easy-goingness may also be migraine co-factors" (79). Is it just in the case of child migraine that even stoicism can be given the negative spin of faking?

Child stoicism can be misinterpreted as painlessness, attempts to pass as easygoing reinterpreted as faking, honest reports as dishonest, and the pain itself as a sign of weakness. Such factors speak more to motives to be silent than any reason to actually admit to migraine as a child. Mary Sheridan writes, "Toddlers have a poor sense of body boundary, and this makes injury or medical treatment even more frightening" (89). Elliot Krane writes, that in particular with repeated pain, which is "especially invisible (e.g. migraine, abdominal pain, chronic ear pain), preschool children cannot understand what's happening" (11). These young children are still struggling to figure out that others can't see their pain, that it's fully up to them to communicate it, so when they do, we should actively listen rather than discourage any further disclosure. This means that "[p]arents need to view their child's pain with different eyes—with the eyes of the child they once were," but if adults did not experience repeated, dysfunctional pain at that age, even this empathy is a challenge (Krane 19). Development also plays a role in this dilemma that needs to be understood by parents, educators, and health-care providers: "Younger children are more likely to think they are having pain because they've done something wrong," which also leads young children who are not in pain to see those in pain as deserving it (Krane 219). Arlene B. Brewster points out that the common child perception of "illness as punishment, feeling that they brought about their illnesses by their own bad deeds, thoughts, or wishes" also discourages coming forward. This and the genuine stoicism they are learning might be enough to cause children to downplay their pain in social settings and only seek help once it is unbearable.

And it's not just in home and school environments that misapplied guilt and migraineur silence/stillness is misinterpreted. Medical doctors, who have no excuse for not knowing any better, contribute to such prejudices. Frank Vertosick writes, "A close friend of mine, a nephrologist practicing in Florida, teases me by saying that migraines are just routine headaches that occur in wimps" (17). His rebuttal is to bring up the case of migraineur Terrell Davis, saying, "All due respects to my Florida friend, but professional football players do not generally qualify as wimps" (18). He also gives this great example about Fred Couples:

> I was watching a recent professional golf tournament, and the golfer who was leading the field almost pulled out during the last round because of his migraine. He struggled through and went on to win, yet he almost traded $700,000 for a chance to go lie down. These examples put some perspective on how bad the pain can be.
>
> (18)

As with the posthumous diagnosing of authors and artists, using "inspiring" examples of migraineurs who overcome the pain is a common device in migraine literature, but the use of athletic narratives in particular reveals a sublimated fear of being cast a runt by focusing on figures whose physical strength already counters such categories by association.

Terrell Davis's story is particularly sensational but reveals how socio-structural factors determine when we respond to migraine with appropriate compassion and respect, and when we do not. The famous Broncos running back was playing in the 1998 Superbowl when he started to get his familiar prodromal symptom, almost complete blindness. He knew an attack was coming (he'd forgotten to take his prophylactic medications), but worse for the moment, he was pivotal to the next play and couldn't see. So he toughed it out and blindly misdirected the other team in a fake handoff. It worked. Davis says, "But now, with the play done and the left side of my head pulsating and throbbing, I needed help right away. . . . I was treated like an emergency-room patient, all kinds of immediate attentions" (1998, 3). Sitting out the second quarter, with oxygen, Migranal nasal spray, and a spell of vomiting, Terrell was ready to play again, an act which became the heroic sports story of the season (the Broncos won). Frank Vertosick emphasizes the validation of migraine pain by the highly publicized episode, stressing that Davis "had to sit out a portion of the [Superbowl] game because of a migraine—imagine the headache that could keep a player out of *that* arena" (18).

In a similar defense, more recent outings of high-profile athletes with migraine have been helpful in gaining recognition of just how debilitating the condition can be, because the "wimp factor" is so obviously misprojected (and hopefully, as a result these prejudices may be questioned). When in April of 2010, the Vikings' wide-receiver Percy Harvin was taken on a stretcher to the hospital after collapsing from migraine at practice, media coverage included dramatic affirmations like "it's a *horrifying* migraine attack" (my emphasis). When in October of 2014, Dolphin left-guard Daryn Colledge had to leave a game for migraine, NBC Sports responded, "Colledge was struggling *mightily* before heading to the locker room" (my emphasis). An unsettling number of examples come from football, like Cardale Jones, an Ohio State University quarterback, who was "rushed to the hospital . . . with severe head pain" in September of 2015 (Endebrock). Usually the severity, reality, and manliness of these attacks are somehow qualified with phrases like "Jones suffered from a *very bad* migraine" (my emphasis, Endebrock). All this indicates some progress in the public profile of migraine, which is at least better understood in the sports community—Miami Heat's Dwayne Wade, one of the top players in the NBA, is very open about his migraine, which he's had since childhood, and he doesn't have to be apologetic when he can't play; he even wears special glasses at practice to reduce glare.[16] Though bylines may sound a bit blaming, as in the November 2015 loss covered as "Hawks, Wade Migraine Too Much for Heat to Overcome," they also dignify the disorder with details from Wade himself: "My vision got blurry. I was having trouble seeing. It just came on. It got me" (Winderman). Wade's descriptions echo those of literary and everyday migraineurs quoted at length here: "[W]hen it wants to come on, it just comes on." Such developments indeed encourage recognizing migraine pain as truly debilitating and also indicate acceptance of certain special needs for a migraineur's alternate abling, but no doubt the heroic interpretations (rather than deeming Davis, Couples, Wade, Harvin, Colledge, or Jones as "wimps") are influenced by issues of gender, athleticism, and age. The kid who needs to sit out part of their little league game for a headache will hardly be hailed as a hero. The child who skips a few exercises at the barre during ballet class is not called a hero either. Terrell Davis got the MVP award.[17]

In his memoirs, *TD: Dreams in Motion*, Davis makes this contrast in treatment between young migraineurs and highly paid athletes very evident:

> People tell me how brave it has been of me to play in these NFL games with classic migraines. Trust me. It's nothing compared to what I endured in high school and college. . . . Of course, it was not like people were willing to give me the same kind of medical attention I get today, when doctors treat each one of my headaches with the care that surgeons usually reserve for organ

transplants. Back then, other than my family and friends, no one really cared who Terrell Davis was or how much pain I was in. I lived with my headaches the way some of my friends lived in poverty. No choice, man.

(62–63)

Only one of the migraineurs I interviewed was ever taken to the emergency room as a minor for rescue palliative medication, and that was when she was a teenager (Goedert, Dee), but each could recall a particularly severe attack that made them question why more extreme treatment was not even considered. Marginalized groups (the young, the poor, and nonwhites) are less likely to be taken seriously with varying degrees of self-rated pain, or adequate medical care is simply not accessible. Tietjen et al. found among adolescents that "in migraine subjects without a strong genetic predisposition, low household-income was a marker of increased prevalence, suggesting a role for environmental risk factors" (28). Else-Karin Grøholt et al. argue, "Children living in low educated, low-income, worker families had approximately a 1.4-fold odds of having pain" (965). Sillanpää and Anttila found that "low economic status of the family, participation in daycare, dwelling in other than a one-family house, and a high number of leisure activities—all independently explained the occurrence of headache in 5-year old children" (1996, 469). Yet, in the hierarchy of pain that exists in the United States, wherein adult pain is treated more than child pain, men's pain is treated more than women's, white patients' pain is more treated than that of nonwhite patients, and of course the wealthy are treated more for pain than their poorer counterparts,[18] often the people who are proven to need it most are getting the least[19] (Thernstrom 167). Walter F. Stewart has even suggested that "[i]n some individuals migraine may cause low income. That is, headache-related disability may seriously disrupt function at work or school. The phenomenon of 'downward' socioeconomic drift has been described in other disabling conditions" (68).

Lower-income patients of all ages, who are less likely to have insurance and more likely to rely upon Medicaid, are already less likely to be treated for migraine. According to a 2010 study,

> The uninsured, and those with Medicaid, receive substandard therapy for migraine, at least in part because they receive more care in emergency departments and less in physician's offices. . . . 5.5 million Americans risk substandard treatment of their migraine and consequent avoidable suffering and disability.

(Wilper et al., 1178)

A 2011 study indicates that one barrier to proper care for children with Medicaid is the lack of accessibility to specialists: for example, in attempts to get an appointment with neurologists, children with private insurance were 43% more likely to get appointments with a neurologist than children with public insurance, and those with public insurance who did succeed at getting appointments averaged a 22-day longer wait (Bisgaier 2324, 2329). A 2014 study found a particular discrepancy in children without private insurance receiving fewer abortive or prophylactic medications for migraine (Mateen 143).

Top sports figures who live with migraine are in most senses the exception to the rule in our cultural neglect of migraine pain, but Terrell Davis hasn't forgotten the challenges of being a child migraineur without access to adequate medical help. He shares stories of denial and abuse that are similar to those of many migraineurs who were children with the attacks. Coaches misunderstood and didn't help. His own father contributed to the misery:

> One time, when Terrell could not read the chalkboard [due to prodromal blindness], the teacher sent him to the office. The principal called Pops to come and get him. At home, Terrell couldn't even hang up his jacket in the closet. Pops yelled at him. "I kept trying, but I couldn't do it," Terrell said. "My depth perception and motor skills were off." Pops tore his belt from his pants, yanked down Terrell's pants, and gave him a fierce whipping.
>
> (Savage 22)

Helen Neal writes that

> among those who develop the highest pain thresholds are battered children[20] and professional football players. . . . [T]he children having learned that screams of pain bring on more punishment, the football players controlling their expressions of pain to stay in the game and keep their jobs.
>
> (42)

If this is true for Terrell Davis, it helps to further indicate the validity of his response to migraine (not that it should be questioned).

The roughness of sports has been directly connected with precipitating migraine attacks. Simply put, we now know that "[h]eadaches are the most common symptom of sport-related concussion" and that "trauma to the head can result in the onset of migraine headaches" (Meehan 104). But this knowledge has been slow in changing public perceptions. In 1972 *The British Medical Journal* published a series of commentaries[21] on "Footballer's Migraine" (referring to soccer, but clearly applying to American football as well). One example comes from a juvenile case:

> A boy of 12 was playing somewhat inexpertly in goal when he was struck on the side of the head by the ball. Within a few minutes he complained of blurred vision and a little later developed numbness in the right hand and difficulty with speech. As this improved, it was followed by severe headache and he was taken to a hospital. . . . He had no previous history of migraine.
>
> (Matthews 326)

Yet W. B. Matthews takes this as evidence that migraine might be an "occupational hazard . . . occurring only when playing football and precipitated by head trauma" rather than reflecting on the danger presented specifically for children (326). He argues instead that "it cannot be known how often a promising career in football or boxing is given up on this account" (327). Such diversions of logic reveal the power of masculine culture over caution. As Judith (Jack) Halberstam points out, the ability to take a beating is culturally valued in the cult of masculinity, as demonstrated by certain formulas in boxing films:

> [T]he masculinity of the boxer is determined not by how quickly he can knock the other guy out but by how many punches the boxer can take without going down himself. In these films, boxing is a trial in which the male body withstands physical assault. . . . [T]he most macho of spectacles is the battered male body, a bloody hunk of ruined flesh.
>
> (274–275)

Such standards may put boys who reject this version of masculinity in a dilemma—enduring pain becomes an imposed ideal, so one must silently endure and let their wounds speak for their toughness. But migraine has no wound to speak.

Even so, stoicism is more likely assumed in males, thus helping to validate their pain reports more than those of females. Martin Pernick explains that "traditional concepts of virility presumed a truly masculine man to be almost impervious to physical pain"; thus, "[w]hen a man feels pain, it is serious" (150). And so, male pain is treated more aggressively than female pain. Dorothea Z. Lack demonstrated that this paradox plays out empirically:

> We found that women received many more prescriptions for minor tranquilizers than men, and that Valium was most often prescribed. Women also received more antidepressants, analgesics, and "other" medications. . . . Men received more narcotics considerably more often than women.
>
> (57)

Joanna Kempner writes that women have to work harder "to present themselves as credible patients. This often translates into an effort to carefully control gender displays. Nobody wants to be viewed as a whiny, weak-willed girl" (xi). Girls with migraine, then, risk being completely overlooked. Socially imposed codes for femininity predefine them as more likely to whine. Consider the assumptions satirized in Hans Christian Andersen's "Princess and the Pea," from which children may learn that girls are hypersensitive and expected to complain of the slightest pain, and the female might be tested to prove it. Unfortunately, the school nurse can't test the veracity of a child's migraine by sticking a pea under her mattress.

Helen Neal writes,

> A child is easier to ignore than an adult. A child cannot take his complaint to the head nurse or to the hospital administrator. A child does not write indignant letters to the editor of the local newspaper revealing the callous treatment he

received in the local hospital. Nor does a child bring consumer action against the hospital for causing his undue suffering.

(168)

Charles Berde et al. write, "Children lack economic power. If adults are unhappy with their postoperative pain management they might not pay their bills" (99). At least they report that "[i]n recent years, more parents have become vocal advocates for their children's pain management" (99). But in schools, medical practice, and within their communities, children are aware of their own silencing—they know they aren't granted the power of a voice. Janet Geddis expresses this awareness when she recalls how debilitating her migraines became in high school: "Things may have been easier on me had I not kept the pain a secret. The majority of my closest friends had no idea. I was suffering. . . . I didn't feel old enough or mature enough to have an illness that had to be taken seriously" (quoted in Laurie Edwards, 73). Far from exaggerating, child migraineurs often suffer silently much more than they complain.

And of course, it is children in the worst conditions who have the least power or resources, as illustrated in migraineur Ishmael Beah's *A Long Way Gone: Memoirs of a Boy Soldier* (2007). Beah, as a child, experienced horrific shock and instability— separated from his family, which he lost then to political violence, swept up into the child-exploiting civil war in his country, Sierra Leone. His case is extraordinary yet alludes to the same silencing and invisibility of migraine experienced by many children:

> I distanced myself from games in the village . . . until my migraines temporarily subsided. I didn't tell anyone what was happening to me. My symptoms weren't mentioned in the morning when the "sergeant doctor" – as civilians called him – lined up children and families for treatment. The sergeant doctor called for fever, cold, and many other illnesses, but he never asked if anyone was having nightmares or migraines. . . . I quietly sat in the corner of the room clenching my teeth, as I didn't want to show my friends the pain I felt from my headache.
>
> (102–103)

Beah's diagnostic details echo with his everyday trauma:

> In my mind's eye I would see sparks of flame, flashes of scenes I had witnessed, and the agonizing voices of children and women would come alive in my head. I cried quietly as my head beat like the clapper of a bell.
>
> (102–103)

Even to a child migraineur who lives safely with family and away from the everyday duress of political violence, erratic sleep[22] can be a strong predictor of migraine activity. But anxiety compounds insomnia, as does Beah's processing of constant trauma through nightmares:

Sometimes I was able to fall asleep briefly, only to be awoken by nightmares. One night I dreamt that I was shot in the head. I was lying in my blood as people hurriedly walked past me. A dog came by and began licking my blood ferociously. The dog bared its teeth as my blood sweetened its mouth. I wanted to scare it away, but I was unable to move. I woke up before it started what I was afraid it was going to do to me. I was sweating and couldn't sleep for the rest of the night.

(102–103)

When he begins daily ingestion of amphetamines, "smoking marijuana, and sniffing brown brown, cocaine mixed with gunpowder," his migraines abate (121). And when the drugs are no longer supplied Beah says,

My hands had begun to shake uncontrollably and my migraines had returned with a vengeance. It was as if a blacksmith had an anvil in my head. I would hear and feel the hammering of metal in my head, and these unbearable sharp sounds made my veins and muscles sour. I cringed and rolled around on the floor by my bed or sometimes on the verandah. No one paid any attention, as everyone was busy going through their own withdrawal stages in different ways.

(140)

Indirectly, the reader can infer Beah's extreme tolerance for pain and his stoicism. In such extraordinary conditions, he is lucky to get medical attention, as when he faints from migraine and awakens in a hospital, or when he punches out windows in a school and gets glass embedded in his skin, a nurse works on removing the shards:

She twisted her face whenever she was removing a piece of glass that was buried deep in my skin. But when she looked at me, I was still. She searched my face to see if I was in pain. She was confused, but continued to gently remove the pieces of glass from my bleeding hand. I didn't feel a thing. I just wanted to stop my blood from flowing.

(141)

Of course I'm not suggesting that Beah's tolerance of pain comes from his frequent exposure to migraine pain—after all, he's numbed by trauma. But such examples speak to how difficult it is to gauge stoicism when the pain is not from visible glass shards but migraine.

You can't judge from self-reports alone whether or not the person in pain is actually downplaying the pain, being as tough as possible. When I asked migraineurs how the disorder may have affected their personalities, the most common answers I heard were "I have a very high tolerance for pain" and then, on some reflection, "I'm more empathetic to the suffering of others." In spite of all I've learned in my research, I found myself sometimes doubting the former, perhaps even projecting on my interview subjects the same prejudices I'd felt against myself since my first attack as a child—maybe they just *think* the pain is worse. Then, in a follow-up interview with Annecy Crockett and her mother, Carrie, the following interchange occurred:

Mother:	"She was throwing up all over the bus, it was terrible."
Daughter:	"I was *not!*"
Mother:	"Oh, right, they had to keep stopping to let you get off and vomit."
Daughter:	"Yeah, but it wasn't *that* bad."
Interviewer:	"How many times did you have to stop?"
Daughter:	"Eight or nine times, but just until I was dry heaving."

I'd taken Annecy's words at face value, overlooking her tendency to downplay her suffering, but in this conversation I realized that we are all subject to downplaying the pain of others—even in the most sympathetic of contexts. Jean Jackson found, in her ethnographic studies of pain clinics, that patients "indicate that they are not quite ready to accept their pain as less organic, less 'real' than they thought. However, they have come to see some of their fellow patients' pain as not entirely organic and real" (1992, 152). All of us, those in pain and those not, need to learn that part of empathy is an ability to read between the lines when it comes to pain reports or the stoic silencing of them. Even for adults who've racked up years of experience with pain and the disbelief of others, this is an ongoing challenge: "Noel Edwards, a migraine sufferer" whose own family stopped believing in his pain, told Jean Jackson, "It's difficult to understand what it's like to have a headache for three years. It's never stopped . . . it's easy to be taken for a hypochondriac" (2005, 340). If an adult, who can aggressively advocate for himself medically, is up against such suspicions, imagine being the migraining child who cannot.

Letty Cottin Pogrebin has written that "[t]hough most of us make exceptions for our own offspring, we do not seem particularly warm hearted towards other people's children" (49). She advises that "[w]e need to bounce our voices off children's silence" (48). And this takes vigilance, active listening, and informed empathy. Marquetta F. Russell copes by imagining "dissolving obstacles." We must "dissolve" trigemony where we can—learn from the suffering, and toughness, of others—an imperative articulated in Jennette Fulda's somber recognition when her head pain became chronic, "There was so much suffering in the world that went unnoticed. Now I could see so many things that used to be invisible. I wasn't sure if I should be grateful for that or not" (107). Some learn empathy through their own pain; the rest of us have to learn by listening and witnessing pain in the stories of others.

Is migraine a spectrum illness, brain disease, (un)healthy impairment, episodic rupture to the bodymind experience, fluctuating invisible disability? Alick Elithorn has called it both a "genetically predetermined disability" and a "recurrent relapsing disability," terms which capture its seemingly ambiguous presence (1969). Most of the migraineurs I interviewed were ambivalent about calling migraine a disability, not because it isn't debilitating, but out of respect for and empathy with those who *appear* to have more limitations. There is also a tendency to be in denial about our own vulnerabilities, as Susan Wendell explains, some "say that they do not consider themselves disabled because 'others are so much worse off than I am.' I think it is sometimes a way of minimizing one's own difficulties in order not to feel frustration, grief, or shame" (27). But if we acknowledge our vulnerabilities, we can open conversations toward greater solidarity with those we perceive as in even greater need of accommodation.

Because migraine ranges on a wide spectrum (from minor to debilitating) and is very common, it too easily escapes politicized attention. Paula Kamen writes that migraine "was too invisible to inspire sympathy, too strangely embarrassing to talk about, and too common to be a disability" (12). But I found, in part from the sense of community I gained in interviewing migraineurs, the immensely empowering experience that disability solidarity fosters—to recognize that each of us share vulnerabilities that can extend our understanding within and to a much larger group of fellow beings, all the while respecting individual difference, self-report, and the diversity of our experiences. We have no choice but to believe and offer support when migraineurs rate their pain as severe, regardless of age.

Though migraine is less common in children than adults, it can be just as debilitating for them. In fact, I agree with Terrell Davis—if severe and/or frequent, it's a far more difficult for children to experience in our culture because of social neglect. Arthur W. Frank argues that

> [p]ain is thus one of the first experiences an ill person has of being cast out. To regain a sense of coherence, in which pain may have to remain a part, the ill person has to find a way back in among those he has become separated from.
> (2002, 31)

A child migraineur's discovery that even her parents cannot stop the pain, are incapable of advocating sufficiently, or in some cases don't even believe it exists, can force a deep existential crisis:

> As adults we also know that pain can usually be treated successfully with drugs or an alternative approach. That is, because we have a vast store of reference, we know there is an end in sight. Young children, however, only know the moment, and imagine the pain will go on forever. The younger the child, the smaller his or her frame of reference, and so the fear of endless pain is more real.
> (Krane 8–9)

Migraine presents serious and unique challenges for children—challenges that could be greatly diminished with heightened cultural awareness. After all, "disability" is framed socially—a construct that pervades individual experience—we can choose as a society to foster coping agency for those experiencing diverse forms of impairment.

Migraine is a trigeminovascular impairment that, due to its invisibility, plays a liminal role in medical practice and disability politics. Child migraineurs occupy an even more marginalized social space that extends to home and school, not for lack of concern, but for the reason that we collectively *will* children through our own denial to be our healthiest demographic—which in the United States is abysmally inaccurate. Those of us who suffer from this condition are not wimps: "The severity of migraines stems from the magnitude of the pain, not from the oversensitivity of the afflicted" (Vertosick 17). Socially, when we are made to feel like runts, we still have power—power to endure, power to express our pain without apology, and power to cope. Voicing authentic legitimacy narratives to validate pain experience is only part of heightening awareness—we have to make others see it, too.

Notes

1 Andrew Levy agrees, writing that "Nietzsche's earthier dreams of Superman . . . stemmed from the desire to rise above some ineffable force holding one down, to beat the enigma of pain through prose and through thought" (130). But mind didn't overcome matter. Among his early treatments were rest, bleedings, and leeches (25–26). Alice Miller stresses the needlessness of his pain, writing that Nietzsche suffered from suppressed rage: "[I]t is no wonder that he suffered continually from severe headaches, sore throats, and rheumatic ailments as a child and especially during his school days. What he was not allowed to say out loud remained active in his body in the form of constant tension" (1990, 84). In a letter dated April 10, 1888, the middle-aged Nietzsche reflected that "There were extremely painful and obstinate headaches which exhausted all my strength. They increased over long years, to reach a climax at which pain was habitual, so that any given year contained for me two hundred days of pain" (519).

2 Loved ones, however, can often tell the migraineur is having an attack by looking at them, although none could articulate what they saw that indicated it. Oliver Sacks describes a visible difference to what he calls "red" and "white" migraines: "[P]atients prone to 'red' migraines tend to be overtly excitable and to flush with anger . . . while other patients prone to 'white' migraines tend to pallor, fainting, and withdrawal reactions in the face to emotional stimuli . . . but no general statement on the subject is applicable to migraine patients in their entirety" (124). I don't know if Hugh Laurie is a migraineur or not, but he does a pretty convincing job of acting out an attack, which he aborts with LSD, in season 2, episode 12 of *House M.D.* (Kaplaw).

3 Andrew Levy writes, "[M]id-migraine, the most twee folk song sounds like death metal turned up to 11," but also he muses "the migraine is not classical, it is not hip-hop, it is definitely punkish – a growl in the guitars, looping feedback and static and then some lo-fi drums, and then a voice, too loud, too jittery, too high, on edge, fast and then faster" (207–208).

4 Oliver Sacks writes, "The literature makes many references to whitening and loss of scalp hair following repeated migraines. The only case suggestive of this, in my own experience, was that of a middle-aged woman who had had very severe, frequent attacks of invariably left-side hemicranias, and in her mid-twenties developed a startling streak of white hair on this side, the remainder of her hair remaining jet-black until many years later" (24).

5 Dr. Haan also explains in print, "diagnosis of migraine is solely and completely based on the narrative of the patient" (2013, 126).

6 Oliver Sacks writes, "It is of more than historical interest that so many authors, from antiquity to the present day, are concerned to present so flattering a picture of the

migraineur. Perhaps one may connect this tendency with the fact that most writers on migraine suffer from migraine" (124).

7 This and the popularity of migraine art may have prompted the common misperception that all auras are visual, when in fact they range from phantom smells, yawning, Reynaud's syndrome, visual disturbance (hallucination to blindness), paralysis, and even in one child case referred to me by Klaus Podoll, auditory hallucinations (13 August 2013).

8 Sacks is, however, probably not too inaccurate when he ties this sense of relief to cyclical depression, though he generalizes too much (40). Migraine is considered comorbid with depression and bipolar states, but that does not mean that relief itself is mania or even euphoria.

9 Think of the Red Queen in *Through the Looking-Glass*, rushing to stay in place. For more on migraine aura with time hallucinations, see Dooley et al. (1990) for six child case studies.

10 Joanna Kempner writes that "The dearth of federal funding means that almost all headache-disorders research is funded by the pharmaceutical industry" (9).

11 Just in case these sound like common sense, I'll explain. First, prophylactic and abortive drugs for migraine attack do not treat the pain, they go as close to the known causes as possible – inhibiting cortical spreading depression, lowering blood pressure, causing vasoconstriction or dilation (depending on timing), or altering convulsive brain patterns. Second, I've been a migraineur for at least 45 years (and had been for 25 when I got this professor's unsolicited advice), and I'm pretty self-educated in advocating for my health care. Like every other person with severe migraine I've ever met, I've tried everything. Pain forces you to do research and give anything a try. Of course food and sleep can be triggers – I didn't need a relative stranger to tell me that. During chronic periods, my lifestyle is hyperdetermined by migraine (and for years was carefully documented in a migraine diary), down to practically everything I eat, and the vigilant regulations I have to impose upon my sleeping habits, so hearing that I wasn't attentive to these issues struck a very sore spot.

12 Menstrual migraine attacks are usually reported as much less severe but more tenacious (long-lasting) and likely to rebound.

13 See Erik Ask-Upmark's "Migraine May Cause Death" and Teri Roberts (dedication, 59–60).

14 This study was conducted through support from Glaxo, for what that counts: "The risk of developing Major Depression Disorder is increased four-fold and Panic disorder twelve-fold for young adults with migraine. Furthermore, children with headache show less social participation and more somatic complaints. In addition, they are less happy at school and even more anxious than the children with no pain" (Langeveld 184).

15 For a more light-hearted fictional version see Phillip Pullman's *The Golden Compass*. The fact that child "battles" can be treated nostalgically speaks to their murky entrenchment culturally. Distinguishing play from bullying can be difficult – both have deep, common cultural roots. Pullman also dips into the more sinister tradition of abandoning and sacrificing children in the medieval tradition of oblation in this novel.

16 These are also helpful for watching TV and wearing in movie theaters, though only partially supported by empirical research (Wilkins et al. 2002, Wilkins et al. 2007). You can just have old prescription glasses shaded red (the best color for reducing glare and flickering effects that may trigger an attack) or purchase special FL41 lenses. One study suggests that "children wearing rose tints" sustained the most reduction in attacks (Good et al. 1991).

17 Of course, much of this congratulatory praise is dependent upon winning. As Joanna Kempner points out, Scottie Pippen's experience with the media reveals quite a contrast: "To this day, whenever sports fans and commentators talk about or interview Pippen, they inevitably turn to the migraine that kept him from helping the Bulls win the 1990 Eastern Conference Championship" (2).

18 Within childhood studies, Anna Mae Duane's and Robin Bernstein's work exposing racial bias in the historic depiction of child pain is necessarily limited to discursive examples, which can lead to conflating pain with all suffering, including "sorrows" (see Duane 7, 17 and Bernstein 61). Patricia Crain writes of this challenge, "The materials that might reveal something about the children in question are naturally difficult to access; there's little in the way of firsthand testimony or narrative of any kind by children in any period" (419). Nonetheless, Duane and Bernstein have raised awareness in the humanities of racial bias in recognizing child pain. Another inequity in pain treatment has been observed geographically: urban hospitals show a "more liberal use of narcotics than the rural hospital" (Schechter et al. 1986, 14).

19 Michael J. Cousins et al. point out that "the gap between deepening knowledge about pain and clinically inadequate treatment is widening – in aggregate, fewer than 50% of patients with acute, chronic, or cancer pain receive adequate relief" (1).

20 Most children, however, are not tough to the pain, nor should they be expected to be. Elsewhere Helen Neal writes, "children's tolerance is generally far below that of adults (athletes manage pain much better than the rest of us)" (101). As mentioned before, Tietjen et al. show that "emotional abuse was associated with severe headache-related disability, allodynia, as well as with earlier age of migraine onset" (35). But "the prevalence of emotional abuse in our population was substantially higher than in other clinic-based and community studies" of non-migraine patients (28).

21 See also A. M. Morris and Michael L. E. Espir et al.

22 Minna Aromaa wrote, in one study, that "[f]atigue and sleep deprivation were the most common triggers of headache" (1731). In another, "Recurrent difficulties in falling asleep at 3 years were also predictive of later headache" and "concentration difficulties, behavioral problems, and unusual tiredness at 5 years were also strong predictors" (25). These studies included nonmigrainous headache.

5 Visibility machines and pain proxies

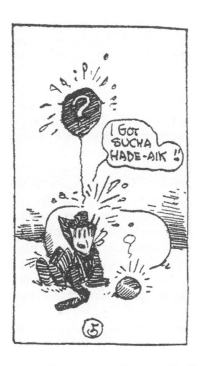

Figure 5.1 © George Herriman. 1920. Courtesy of Fantagraphics Books (fantagraphics.com)

Patients who experience prolonged periods of episodic or chronic pain often feel most alienated by its invisibility. Jean Jackson writes, "Although some people with visible marks would prefer a concealable condition, chronic pain sufferers sometimes bemoan the invisibility of their pain, saying they would prefer a more visible—even though also more stigmatized—condition," because visible impairments are recognized and treated as real, so they can at least be dealt with head-on (2005, 341). Two literary anecdotes exemplify methods by which visible impairments (or scars left by them) can be directly demarginalized for children. In the first, coming from Deborah Ellis in *No Ordinary Day* (2011), a homeless orphan in Kolkata meets other patients in a leprosy ward of a hospital who are already visibly marked by the disease, and, based on the lore of her upbringing, the child thinks they are "monsters." But one of them tells her "Look at me until you see me" (135). Valli breaks her habitual uncomfortable stare and down-turned eyes to see beyond her fear into understanding what is a surface trait, the scars of past disease:

> And something happened. I stopped seeing the caved-in nose. I stopped seeing the damaged eye with its drooping eyelid and milky-looking eyeball. And I stopped seeing the stubs of fingers. Instead I saw the face of the woman who had brought me a good cup of tea. I saw little lines around the corners of her eyes. I saw kindness in her smile. I saw a woman who was stubborn and hard working and did not want to hurt me.
>
> (135–136)

Ellis both visually depicts a healthy thriving body scarred by past disease and gets beyond the biases against visible difference through refamiliarization in this interaction. In contrast, consider R. J. Palacio's *Wonder* (2012), in which the narrator, Auggie, a boy born with facial structural abnormalities does quite the opposite—redirecting familiarization. On introducing himself he tells the reader, "I won't describe what I look like. Whatever you're thinking, it's probably worse" (3). Palacio waits until a good 80 pages later to let Auggie's sister, the second narrator, describe Auggie's face. The literary technique is the opposite of Ellis's, but the effect on the reader is similar. We look beyond a body to "see" the person. The latter is an ideal but evasive and impractical strategy for face-to-face meetings. The former exemplifies the seeming paradox that by looking closely, and beholding visible bodies otherwise marginalized by culture (even as images), we can transcend the isolating and ablest norms that prevent us from seeing beyond visible difference.

Elizabeth Wheeler points out that though oversimplifying,

> *Wonder* plays out the competing concepts of disability named and analyzed in disability studies: the social model, the medical model, and what we might call a monster model. The novel recapitulates the history of disability representation. It moves beyond damaging ideas, shifts the weight of these ideas off August's shoulders, and leaves room for a more humane model of disability.
>
> (339)

By depicting such a layered perspective the novel directly addresses biases that young readers may recognize they have held (like Valli, thinking of different others as monsters, learning through medicalized explanations that difference makes sense, coming to understand the negative impact of socially neglecting needed accommodation). No one model unites impaired persons or fully educates those who are in their current embodiment nonimpaired, but multiple perspectives may provide a discursive equivalent of "sustained looking." Rosemarie Garland-Thomson demonstrates throughout *Staring: How We Look*, that

> [w]hen people with stareable bodies . . . enter into the public eye, when they no longer hide themselves or allow themselves to be hidden, the visual landscape enlarges. Their public presence can expand the range of the bodies we expect to see and broaden the terrain where we expect to see such bodies.
>
> (9)

Visibility challenges thoughtless and passive acceptance of damaging norms. In this sense, visualizing "disability" can be affective, but what if impairments are undetectable, and the uncomfortable stares and averted eyes are replaced with a complete lack of recognition? In this case we have to make suffering seen before we can recognize it.

Petra Kuppers argues in her scholarly work and performance for imperatively making visible any impairment which is culturally invisible (be it exposing suffering and the impairment itself, or celebrating alternative ability). She writes, "By structuring the visibility machine of performance, we intervene in the violations of the 'medical stare' at different bodies" (2005, 148). Early attempts at creating this visibility were flawed by condescension, overstating difference, and focusing less on impaired persons or disability than on doctors who "cured" them. Kuppers characterizes a shift in approaches to creating visibility, in contrast to efforts like those of Jean Martin Charcot (1825–1893) in the 1870s who staged the "hysterical fits" of patients:

> [T]he contemporary situation of disabled people with invisible impairments can still echo this representational past. . . . [But] if Charcot was intent on creating visible discourses for mental difference, contemporary disability artists struggle with the "undoing of fixities and categorical differences."
>
> (2005, 152)

Categories that enabled solidarity in the first place become suspect in this paradigm.

Medical accounts are inadequate when it comes to culturally dismantling stereotypes, so one objective of disability activism has been to replace "medical diagnostic labeling and its mechanism of grouping, erasing patient's specificity" with an emphasis on "individual specificity and nonnormative singularity" (Kuppers 2007, 148). But intersubjective understanding is particularly difficult when it comes to dysfunctional pain. No one can see it. Elaine Scarry writes, "The difficulty of imagining others is shown by the fact that one can be in the presence of another person who is in pain and not know that the person is in pain. The ease of remaining ignorant of another person's pain even permits one to inflict it and amplify it in the body of the other person while remaining immune oneself" (1998, 41). Chronic neuropathic pain is especially easy to misunderstand, writes David Morris: "Its relative invisibility gives chronic pain a feature that makes it both insidious and almost unique." In contrast, "[w]hat AIDS, cancer, tuberculosis, leprosy, madness, and other representative illnesses share is a graphic power to seize the imagination" (66). Former surgeon general (and migraineur) C. Everett Koop explained this misunderstanding partly as a result of unperceivable consequences, namely, fatality:

> You almost have to die of something in order to get the attention that the disease process deserves in the American health system. . . . That's why AIDS, which [was] 100 percent fatal, attracted so much attention. People could understand that. Migraine is 100 percent nonfatal.
>
> (Morris 66)

Even though, as Morris points out, migraine is "the vastly more common" affliction (66), and, I might add, *is* fatal in the rare cases of migraine-induced stroke, dominant ideologies dismiss migraine as "just a bad headache." Of course, migraine has never had the political visibility of AIDS hard-won by queer and disability activists in the 1980s and early 1990s, which made its then-staggering fatality highly visible to the public, pharmaceutical industry, medical researchers, and policy makers.

As part of an effort to correct these misunderstandings through the "graphic power" of visibility machines, joining the tradition of expressing the experience through migraine art, is an emerging genre of medical comics,[1] some of which focus on migraine. Much has been written on the suitability of comics as a medium for articulating "disabled" experience and educating readers about it—some comics artists have proven that their medium is even ideal for visualizing invisible disability and pain in particular (see Freedman). As is well-documented, comics have an inherent edge in cutting through the counterproductive narrative dismissal that socially emerges surrounding invisible disability—they have the potential to disrupt the medical and normative gaze by making individual experience more sympathetically visible and comprehensible as alternatively abled. Susan Squier writes that "works of graphic fiction and narrative demonstrate the power comics have to move us beyond the damaging discourse of developmental normalcy into a genuine encounter with the experience of disability" (86). They also have the unique power of promoting higher visibility and empowerment through redefined agency.

First, by meeting child readers in a medium that already appeals, comics can impart positive vicarious experience. Gerard Jones suggests as much in his *Killing Monsters: Why Children Need Fantasy, Super Heroes, and Make-Believe Violence* in his treatment of comics in general, finding therapeutic value in comic book heroes like Superman:

> I found that for preschoolers his one great power was simply being *above pain*. Pain is a central issue for young children – wondering how bad it will be, how to avoid it, how to be brave when it's inevitable – and Superman being attacked and defeating his foes is a comforting demonstration that one can pass through it and come out happy on the other side.
>
> (222)

Relevantly, Nathan Speer told me that when he was old enough to use triptans, "Imitrex made me feel like Superman." He was not expressing some kind of drug-induced euphoria (triptans don't affect mood or even make one feel drugged up— that's part of their appeal) but the relief from the demoralizing lack of control that comes with chronic pain. Of course, I've been arguing that one part of the sometimes necessary capitulation to using medications is that they can bring a migraineur back in control over the pain, but his identification of such a feeling with superheroes also speaks to the power of comics as a medium for promoting agency.

As Bert Hansen points out, however, initial comics efforts to educate about disability are reduced depictions to hero worship of doctors and indulgence in "cure theories," which may have been partly motivated by the perceived need to contrast the "dominant image of a scientist" as "a wild-eyed, white-coated, ego-tistical maniac" found in earlier superhero comics (182). For example, the heavy pressure to not only *fit* the norm but *look* it is reinforced in a PSA (public service announcement) on polio from a 1942 issue of *True Comics*, in which one char-acter protests "We can't believe you've ever had infantile, Phil! Why, you're just like us!" In the comic, normative marginalizing implicitly hinges on visibility. Pedagogical comics and public service announcements for children demonstrate an early awareness of comics' potential for disability awareness, though flawed with condescension, as seen in a vintage PSA reprinted in Judy and Paul Karasik's *The Ride Together: A Brother and Sister's Memoir of Autism in the Family.* The one-page PSA titled "The Invisible Handicap!" depicts the bullying of a learning-impaired child by another student, who calls him "Dopey" and "a real weirdo," prompting the teacher to explain,

> You're right – something *IS* wrong with him. You wouldn't have acted that way if he were blind and lame. . . . Something you could see. But this new boy happens to have a handicap that's invisible – damage to part of the brain.
>
> (72)

The comic makes his invisible impairment visible through depicting the child's art-work in class as less skillful than that of the others his age, resolving the bullying with the other children shown later behaving in a supporting manner toward the child's efforts (but of course patronizing, like the teacher). Consciously modeling comics as means of promoting disability visibility is the inclusion of the invisibly impaired character's artwork within the comic. This sort of effort would eventually become a standard device in far more sensitive and artistically sophisticated work in which children with invisible illness are depicted as privately engaged in art therapy. David Small does this in *Stitches* (48–49), and Katie Green uses the device[2] in her 2013 comic on anorexia nervosa, *Lighter Than My Shadow* (161). The benefit of visualization by simultaneously imagining oneself as both subject and spectator of chronic illness has been reaffirmed by empirical research. Michael Rich et al. have studied how teens' "visual narratives of their illness experiences" help them to not only express their needs to those around them but contribute to improved quality of life (155).

Certainly demonstrating pedagogical uses of this potential is the Medikidz series explaining a long list of illnesses and disabilities, which are peer-reviewed by medical doctors and relatively well-written for didactic comics (if one can overlook the fat jokes). Sarah Birge highlights the comic-form's ability to represent individual experience, which Medikidz takes advantage of by producing "Superhero Adventure[s] inside the Human Body":

> Although a visual medium might not initially seem most appropriate for representations of disabilities that are often termed "invisible" (because they cannot immediately be read by looking at a person), comics are able to represent aspects of disability that [verbal] text alone cannot, such as the crucial importance of embodiment in the lived experiences of people with disabilities. . . . Comics' ability to represent complex interactions of emotions, thoughts, movements, and social relationships creates a promising opportunity for remedying the inadequacy of many contemporary representations.
>
> (no pagination)

Perhaps most relevant to my argument is *Medikidz Explain Chronic Pain* (as of yet there is not a Medikidz comic on migraine, though they tell me they are working on it). And yet, the Medikidz focus on the invisibility of pain even within panels (showing pain simply with flaring words, "pain"), where a neural messenger has to report the existence of the very pain they are discussing. A cute, sad-eyed messenger explains to a child touring the human body to learn of the condition, "I know I look super adorable and awesome on the outside, but inside I'm hurting." The lack of witnessing causes distress on top of the actual pain—the burden of proof is entirely placed upon sufferer report. As further silencing, the Medikidz comics, which usually focus on child characters coping with illness, with titles about ADHD, cancer, AIDS, epilepsy, asthma, diabetes, and even juvenile arthritis and glaucoma, have only a few titles focused on adult characters, implying that child readers only need to understand these impairments, such as breast cancer and Parkinson's, as something that will affect adults they know, rather than children.

The chronic pain title, "What's Up with Moira's Grandad?" is one of these, and avoids mentioning that children, too, can have dysfunctional pain. This fact is rarely addressed in kids' comics and is only directly graphically addressed in one self-published picture book by migraineur Gretchen Rautman, *My Secret: Me and My Body's Pain,* where she addresses her readers: "Do you have a secret like me? What part of you hurts? Is it your head like me?" Her book explains, in very accessible terms, the double bind of dysfunctional pain for children: "It can be even scarier / When you can't see the pain."

Pain needs a witness, but witnessing requires visual cues. In her essay "Among School Children," Elaine Scarry describes seeing a group of seven-year-olds in a museum selecting paintings with visible wounds as the best representations of pain. Scarry overheard a teacher leading a school class in the Philadelphia Museum of Art with the instructions, "'Now children, I want you to go into the next room and sit in front of the painting that has the most physical pain in it'. . . . Half of the children sat huddled together on the floor beneath Rubens's *Prometheus Bound*; the other half . . . sat silently beneath Pacecco de Rosa's *Massacre of the Innocents* (11). Both paintings show not only blood and wounds, but the physical cause of injury: "depicted are both the agent of the injury (the raptor) and body damage (the exposed organ)" or "swords flash and babies bleed" (11). In her analysis, Scarry realizes that pain is easily perceived with visible wounds, disbelieved without them. She observes via Thomas Szasz that "so much is physical pain felt as mutilation that patients sometimes do physically mutilate their bodies in order to bring the actual body image 'up to date' with felt experience" (14). In either case the visible wound/scar becomes the legitimate site of recognized pain.

This phenomenon enhances appreciation of David Small's focus on his surgical scar in his comics memoir, *Stitches* (see figure 5.2). As a child he is lied to about his cancer, operated on without consent, and loses his voice for a period of time. As a patient neither honestly informed by nor listened to by the adults around him, the young David understands that his only language is "getting sick." But Ariela Freedman points out that Small uses the wound and its scar as the voice of pain: "The scar is presented first horizontally, and then vertically, in a double exposure: in its horizontal aspect it resembles a mouth sewn into silence. And the wound seems to speak. . . . The scar speaks to us as well" (393). The implications of this wound-focus for comics are considerable and well-demonstrated in sudden moments of blunt violence in comics such as Greg Fiering's *Migraine Boy* (see figure 5.3). When viewers refer to certain comics (or film) as "graphic," they mean something beyond the obvious, literal observation of their visual mediums. The term becomes synonymous with "explicit"—often referring to the blood and guts seen (or in the case of sexuality, body parts)—in short, making our insides visible on the outside.

The International Association for the Study of Pain defines pain as "[a]n unpleasant sensory and emotional experience associated with actual or potential tissue damage, or *described in terms of such damage*" (my emphasis; quoted in Schott 210).

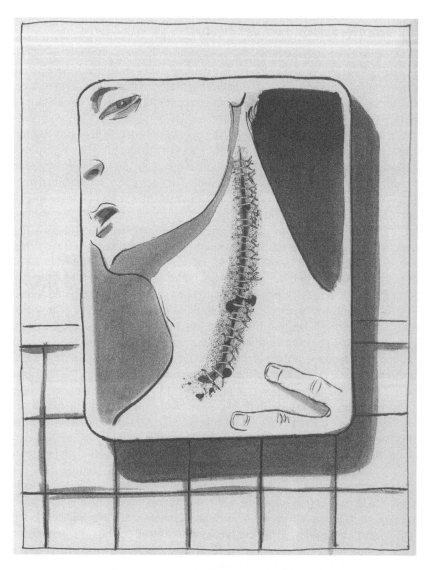

Figure 5.2 From *Stitches: A Memoir*, by David Small. © 2009 David Small. Used with permission of W.W. Norton & Company, Inc.

In the mass of available images from migraine art, migraineurs demonstrate an awareness of the need to show a wound, or at least an offending, visible weapon that can explain their pain. As early as 1830, George Cruikshank would illustrate his "The Headache" not only through an agonized (but somewhat comic) face on the sufferer but more importantly through six small demons who stab his head with

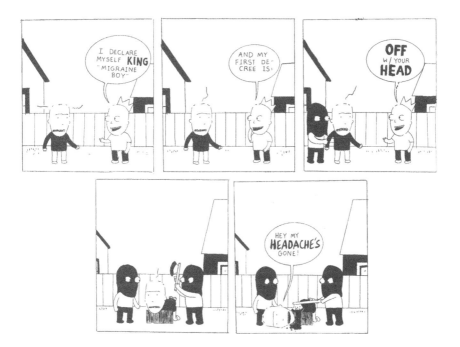

Figure 5.3 Greg Fiering, *Migraine Boy*, 2004. Reprinted with permission of the artist.

a pincer, corkscrew, and oversized mallet, and blow a horn right into his ear, resembling child migraine art discussed in the previous chapter. Knowing this broader context highlights the originality of *H Day* (2010), in which migraineur Renée French (who writes for children under the penname Rainy Dohaney) resists the common tropes yet overcomes the obstacle of visualizing pain through utilizing wordlessness, separate points of view, connecting them with overlapping imagery and theme, externalizing focalization, and promoting reader-identification through an empathetic yet buffered representation of suffering. As such a comprehensive departure, it deserves detailed close reading here to consider new means of promoting visibility and coping.

H Day is a wordless book on migraine experience that follows the phases of a migraine attack in segments called "stages," each double spread containing a representational rendering of a migraineur throughout an attack on the left-hand side, while on the right we enter the migraineur's imagination to experience that character's (and French's own) coping visualizations. In her interview with *USA Today*'s Whitney Matheson, French has explained, "As the headache is happening on the left, the stuff on the right is happening inside his head." French's approach is multidimensional in that it strives to indicate internal causes as well as abstract representations for the holistic experience through her migraine-scape. While admitting the impossibility of adequately depicting the pain, she explains,

> [T]he ones [drawings] on the left to me sort of represent the pain. I know it's not stabbing in my head. It's [the drawing is] not as extreme as what it feels to have a migraine, but the drawings of the person on the bed with the stuff on his head and then strapped to the bed . . . that's kind of to me like illustration of the migraine. I was trying to get at it when you're inside of the headache more.
>
> (Matheson)

As if answering Andrew Levy's call for "an inside language," French has found one of images and space, which allows her to downplay suffering rather than settling on the standard migraine tropes, thus creating an original and individualized experience. Whereas most migraine art depicts auras (what the migraineur sees) or violent wounding (what the viewer must imagine to approximate what the migraineur experiences), French's text depicts how a migraineur might appear during an attack (trying to disappear into the quiet space of the bed) and also what one migraineur *imagines* seeing to distract his mind from that suffering (see figure 5.4).

Viewers of all ages seem to have trouble understanding that a painless but visible wound isn't painful, or the opposite, that an invisible pain is real. This connection between visibility and empathy explains the profound impact of David Beauchard's *Epileptic* (2005), in which he not only visually represents his brother's grand-mal seizures but makes the invisible suffering of his brother and family also visible through concrete, externalizing symbols. It is through the visibility of

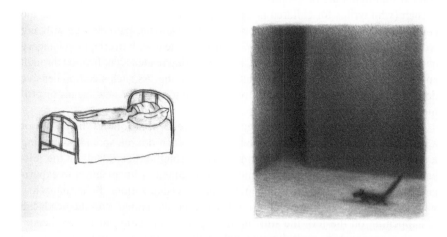

Figure 5.4 Renée French, *H Day*, 2010. Reprinted with permission of the artist.

suffering that we as readers can learn compassion and understanding. *Epileptic* has by now become a touchstone text in proving that comics are capable of circumventing the byzantine narratives of dismissal that surround invisible disability. As Frank Cioffi has argued, graphic medical

> works imitate and replicate the experience of being ill – its frightening, unpredictable out-of-control elements – they also demonstrate that experiences overlap only rarely, for illness and pain are ultimately and always . . . as individual as each reader's experience of a text, as much one's own as pain itself.
>
> (186)

Ariela Freedman adds that "because comics employ both word *and* image, they can try to bridge the internal and external representation of pain" (382). Beauchard exploits all these strengths of the medium without generalizing about disability or promoting a generalizing interpretation.

Migraine and epilepsy are often related as non-neurotypical experiences which involve remarkably similar auras that are invisible to the bystander. Epilepsy is invisible but always on the cusp of visibility, if a seizure should occur—in fact, the primary concerns of children's books on epilepsy tend to hinge on visibility, whether through the exposure of a public episode (as in Patricia Hermes's *What If They Knew?* and Laurie Lears's *Becky the Brave*) or perception as an ontological rupture (as in Thomas Bergman's *Moments That Disappear*). Migraineurs and epileptics are "neurological wild children," as James Berger has dubbed those with access to atypical prelingual perception. Certainly the wealth of attention to the auras of epileptics and migraineurs suggests this fascination with atypical visualizations. Migraine, however, is rarely detectable in any *outwardly* visible manner, almost always requiring narrative explanation, in the same manner as the larger category of neuropathic pain. In the case of migraine, even during attacks the migraineur's posture most likely would not suggest readable pain to those unfamiliar with the sufferer's personality—the complete surrender to stillness and withdrawal from any and all sensory stimulation might look to an outsider a bit like apathy, fatigue, or even relaxation. Yet French overcomes that representational challenge, and, like Beauchard, admirably resists overdependence upon narrative or reducing migraine to a metaphor for something else.

Metaphor can be useful diagnostically, because the similarities of tropes enable identifying with a group similarly impaired, but it can also buffer empathy or misfire completely, as in the figurative projection of pain discussed in chapter 3, when justifying "mercy" killing to put one "out of his pain" (something frequently said when euthanizing animals). Marc Singer explains that comics can counter the slipperiness of such tropes:

> [B]ecause they operate through visual as well as verbal narratives, comics also offer a largely unrecognized opportunity to bypass the master tropes of figurative language. From their inception, comics have denoted otherwise

abstract concepts without resorting to metaphor or metonymy, representing ideas, experiences, and desires through tropes that attempt, however provisionally, to ignore or undo the symbolic deferral of meaning that accompanies all language.

(274)

This potential enables comics artists to concretely represent impaired experience as embodied in the individual without, necessarily, depending upon language.

A unique subjective experience migraineurs often try to articulate is the particular difficulty of distracting one's mind from head pain, seemingly because of its proximity to the intense concentration of sensory input (eyes, ears, nose). French explains in her Strand bookstore talk, "[I]t's unlike a pain in your leg or pain in your arm . . . you can't really separate yourself from it." Perhaps for this reason French did not settle for one sequence representing the impaired experience as an externalized abstract. Elaine Scarry mentions pain "in both medical advertisements and the visual arts as a turning of the body inside out" (1994, 14). French, likewise, turns the migraine inside out[3] in her more representational left-hand renderings. Layered with the right-hand sequences, these indicate what it must look like, what it might feel like, and what might be imagined at the same time—bodyscape and mindscape.

The ubiquitously cited theme of Elaine Scarry's *The Body in Pain* is that pain is word-breaking[4] and world-breaking: "Physical pain does not simply resist language but actively destroys it, bringing about an immediate reversion to a state anterior to language, to the sounds and cries a human being makes before language is learned" (4). Compatible with this "reversion to pre-language," comics on invisible disability promise that art, in response, is world-making.[5] French utilized a wordless format both out of frustration and as a way to overcome the linguistically isolating experience of migraine. In her interview with Tim O'Shea, French explained (ironically, quite well in words), that "a migraine whites out pretty much everything except for your head. I mean, your head becomes the center of everything." The comics artist can circumvent the demand for compulsory narrative, or even the dependence upon words themselves for expressing pain. Whereas some wordless texts, like those of Lynd Ward or Eric Drooker, are nonetheless bursting with sound, French's *H Day* is oppressively silent. This is appropriate to the experience of invisible pain, as David Morris has indicated, "Even the inventive McGill-Mezack Pain Questionnaire reduces the patient's experience of pain to a mere seventy-eight words. . . . Chronic pain opens on an unsocial, wordless terrain where all communication threatens to come to a halt" (73). Like pain therapy that involves imagining rolling all of your pain into a ball and rolling it away from your body (Scarry 2006, 13), French both shows a body in pain and then opens a door to a "wordless terrain" that provides a distraction, or ideally, an escape.

Immanuel Kant's strategy for ignoring his painful gout was "to concentrate all his might on one object, no matter what. . . . Through this method he was so successful in banishing his pain that in the morning he sometimes wondered whether he had simply imagined it" (Morris 7). As mentioned earlier, this may not be so easy during a migraine attack, when concentration only stimulates more pain because concentration usually engages the crisis points of migraine through the senses and facial muscles. Nonetheless, distraction is a primary coping method taught especially to child migraineurs, who are usually considered too young for abortive medication. Short-circuiting the senses by concentrating on an internal world seems to work for French, her migraine protagonist, and dog hero. And one way she circumvents language, and even tight sequentiality, is through juxtaposing an outer point of view with an inner spatialization ("narratives" that, like those of Maurice Sendak or John Burningham, are separately paced). Of course there is sequential plot—the phases of a migraine on the left (prodrome, attack, and postdrome) and the binding by and escape from pain that the dog experiences on the right—but in *H Day*, it is the juxtaposition of perspectives that conveys clues to making sense of the text as a whole.

Susan M. Squier points out that comics are ideal for layering perspectives:

> Rather than leaving the disabled person unable to narrate or represent his full experience, . . . comics make that narrative most fully possible because they include its pre-verbal components: the gestural, embodied physicality of disabled alterity in its precise and valuable specificity.
>
> (85–86)

Whereas in *Epileptic*, David Beauchard uses externalizations (monsters and ornate emotion lines) from his brother's body to represent his experience of seizures, French actually takes us into the imaginary space she visualizes during a migraine attack so that the reader can vicariously experience a coping perspective. The left-hand narrative represents migraine from an outsider's perspective, then the right-hand view doubles over it to present a view from within a migraineur's perspective. French (2013) has said:

> I'd been doing line drawings and diagrams of the inside of heads, sort of diagrams of the pain that comes with a migraine, and . . . I decided to try to draw the stuff I visualize when I've got a headache (the city drawings), the diagrams progressed into the sequence that is in the book (the bed drawings).

The reader sees a clinical progression on one hand, but on the other is invited to enter a space created from pain.

This migraine-scape is unique in the context of prolific migraine art, which usually represents aura or pain, without distracting imagined spaces for the viewer to visit as vicarious embodiments. Perhaps French's technique is even unique within comics. Stephen E. Tabachnick writes, "As Beauchard's invisible-become-visible monsters and the prevalence of dreams informs us . . . [w]e do not need long prose descriptions of how a seizure actually looks, because in *Epileptic* we see seizures in the form of his brother's face and posture" (106). But "[w]e never see what Jean-Christophe sees when he seems to be transported to another world during a seizure" (107). Beauchard does, however, depict battle scenes in great detail, "leaving it to the reader to make the precise connection between those scenes and the family's situation. Yet the connection between the public and the personal is always implied" (109). In contrast, French shows pain both seen and seeing, providing a double agency, but, like Beauchard, she leaves it to the reader to connect the vistas of *H Day*. The presumed effect is to encourage more empathy on the part of the reader comprehensively and quickly. Neuroscientist V. S. Ramachandran even suggests that comics aid more immediate mental processing: "[T]he visual metaphor is probably understood by the right hemisphere long before the more literal-minded left hemisphere[6] can spell out the reasons" (237). By seeing both the migraineur and his migraine-scape, one can more readily comprehend his impaired and coping perspectives. Compared with prose accounts, in which internal narration effects greater intimacy, in the depiction of invisible pain, a simultaneous detachment and disclosure might be necessary.

Consider the concepts of "stopping," "staying," and "doubling" practiced in medicine. Elaine Scarry explains that attending to wounds and pain require very different interaction—for the former, medical personnel must "stay" against the natural reaction to turn away from the weight of empathy (2006, 18), but to treat pain one must engage the subjective experience of the person in pain (2006, 23). Doctors may find themselves needing to "stop" somewhere between clinical objectivity and emotionalism to best treat pain. E. Vegni et al. argue that because of "pain which is not sufficiently understandable in biological terms," doctors face the dilemma of either detaching from patients to the point of inadequately dealing with pain or identifying so much that "the only solution is denial and an escape route" (21, 23). I believe French's artistic choices spring from and perfectly address the challenge of depicting and perceiving pain by suspending the reader in this balanced state of buffered stopping. *H Day* exemplifies the mental process Scarry describes in *Resisting Representation*: "Because pain subverts a person's consciousness of any external world, inside and outside surfaces seem to change places" (32). One resulting solution used in pain clinics is to "double" up on medical personnel—to enable concentrating on each perspective, subjective (inside) and observable (outside). In her representation, French "doubles" perspectives through a bifurcated double spread, as well as using connective imagery and theme between the facing pages.

French's separate but loosely linked narratives provide this "doubling" of perspectives to the reader. They are also visually and conceptually connected. Take, for example, the introductory pages, which precede the "stages" of the attack and lead the reader briefly into the doubling technique with a seemingly single point of view. The first five pages of images appear only on the right, and they are extremely literal and straightforward, at first, as an objective observer might clinically follow the process. We see a (trigeminal?) nerve wrapped in its myelin sheath and vessels, enlarged within the outline of a head like an emphatically disproportioned biological or medical illustration. In the following pages it unwraps as if dissected, with an almost technical instructiveness. But on page 5, the nerve appears emerging from a surface that can only (in my mind) be read metaphorically— like the surface of water, and indeed on the next page we see what appears to be a spouting pipe in the sea (see figure 5.5). The immediate connection for me is to read this pipe as an abstract expression of the intense vasoconstriction and sudden vasodilation that precedes (and at least partially causes the pain of) the migraine attack. It also makes me ask, which was it all along—nerve or blood vessel? Conflating the two actually reflects a long-standing debate about whether migraine is triggered primarily by a neural or vascular dysfunction (though the current consensus is neural). It also introduces the doubling process that will begin with stage 1 and become the model for how to read each subsequent double spread of the story proper.

Doubling points of view in split-perspective double spreads, French continues building possible stories from the attack's process (prodrome/aura, full attack, postdrome), paired with seemingly disconnected elements on the right-hand side:

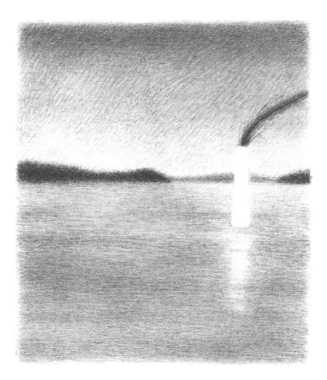

Figure 5.5 Renée French, *H Day*, 2010. Reprinted with permission of the artist.

ants invading spaces, swarming despair, people running from an airborne threat and falling off a building, their dead shapes on the ground also invaded by ants and then turning into vague white sinews. Some of these mysterious images are clarified in French's Strand bookstore signing talk, in which she discusses, among many other things, the ant invasion she experienced in her California home, and the fact that once when she was wetting a cloth in her kitchen to put on her fore-head during a migraine attack, ants got on the towel and her hand, and so they became a part of her inner migraine distraction-imaging, which eventually entered her dreams. Ants and the brain/nerve mechanisms sketched in so much greater detail are the attacking, invading, forces.

We know that visualizing the pain is important to imagining the pain of oth-ers, especially when the cause is concretized as a weapon: "[A] weapon is an object that goes into the body and produces pain; as a perceptual fact, it can lift pain and its attributes out of the body and make them visible" (Scarry 2006, 16). But the epistemological challenge of migraine is its lack of visualizable cause, which explains the plethora of migraine art, like Migraine Boy's in figure 5.6, that is necessarily abstract: "The objectless pain arouses anxiety that focuses on the agent threatening the organism" (Emminghaus, 132). In the case of neuropathic and dysfunctional pain, what is the threatening agent? Migraine seems to compel pictorial renderings which also reveal the impossibility of expressing pain any way but analogically as an attack from outside the body—perhaps even more so

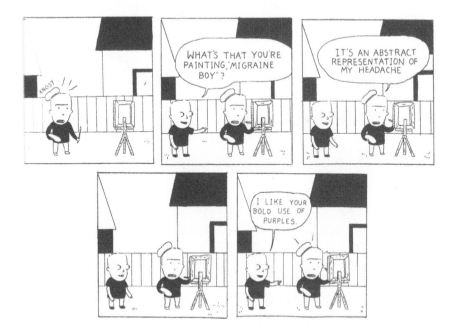

Figure 5.6 Greg Fiering, *Migraine Boy*, 2004. Reprinted with permission of the artist.

because an external cause is rarely detectable (unless you are recognizing tellingly called "triggers").

Wolf B. Emminghaus et al. write, "The most objectless sensory modality is that of pain. Pain also conveys an impression of bodily reality and of the body as a container of experience" (132). Likewise, many since have agreed with Elaine Scarry's well-known premise that "[i]t is precisely because it takes no object that it, more than any other phenomenon, resists objectification in language" (5). Tobin Siebers, in a counter-consideration entitled "In the Name of Pain," demonstrates how the unrootedness and invisibility of pain as a concept can lead to sinister oppression (2010, 184). Petra Kuppers puts an empowering spin on the issue. Whereas for many the supposed wordlessness and objectlessness of pain leaves it inexpressible yet infinitely projectable, Kuppers concludes that "this problem at the empty heart of representation, of focusing pain in language . . . excites the imagination and demands the work of signification" (2007, 76). At any given time in *H Day*, many different images may represent pain to the reader—the swarm cloud, the ants, the white expanding shapes, and even the dog hero—demonstrating all of these features.

But if we take themes which carry over from both the left- and right-hand flow of images as an indication of their multiple or shared meanings, this doubling helps us to linger over their more complicated inter-significance. The ants and the migraine have one very important quality in common, one that is emphasized by French's title—they are both *attacks*, invasions of body and space. French tells Spurgeon, "It's sort of an end of the world book, that migraine book. It's people being attacked by these clouds and dying. All of these people falling off the building and dying. There's only one survivor: the dog." Again, stressing the aggressive, almost violent nature of her subject, French is, whether deliberately or not, taking a stance that is extremely important to debates within disability politics. If migraine is an attack, is it a part of the migraineur's identity or an invasion imposed from outside the migraineur's self-determined identity? This is a very loaded issue, as the former response could essentialize the migraineur and the latter could imply that the migraineur is a victim. Indeed, the common expression "headache sufferer" carries this connotation of passivity in the face of essentialism.

When Scarry observes children selecting visual representations of pain, she differentiates between "actual agent" and "imagined agent," neither of which refers to those suffering, but the pain itself and weapons used to inflict it. Vegni et al. stress, in their argument for necessary detachment in the medical treatment of pain, that "there is a subtractive component, the pain is 'taken away' from the patient and the subject takes on a passive role" (20). In his analysis of online migraine communities and information websites, Georg Marko concludes that

> headache sufferers seem to conceive of themselves, in relation to their condition and to their environment, in terms imposed by medicine and institutional healthcare rather than offering alternatives highlighting the subjective experience of the condition and an agentive approach to it.
>
> (270)

Throughout her book on migraine, Joanna Kempner details some of the ideological underpingings (especially sexism and biological determinism) that complicate agency and resilience for migraining subjects, expressing the crux as resulting from the role of the brain in their disorder:

> Biological explanations of illnesses of the brain do not insulate the person from responsibility for that illness in the same way that disorders of other organs might. This is because in Western countries, the brain has become the organ of personhood.
>
> (101)

Again we are reminded of the trap trigemony sets as well. Clearly agentive models are more resilient than passive victimhood, but the "pride" model (affirming impairment within the normal range of human conditions or celebrating deviation to diversify the norm, as in "queer" and "crip" models) can also be misprojected in essentializing migraineurs as agents of their own suffering.

The problem is that both lines of reasoning, embracing migraineur identity and seeing oneself as a victim of migraine attacks, can be used to marginalize migraineurs—even agentive arguments can be turned around to implicitly blame the migraineur who gets attacks in spite of advocating for their health aggressively through alternative therapies, homeopathic and allopathic medicine, diet, lifestyle, and education. If you are the agent, this idea implies that you are also responsible for your pain. You simply aren't doing enough to stop it. Even more important to note is that just saying that someone has agency does not make attacks cease, and wanting them to cease is not simply an acceptance of "cure" theories that make us drugged-up dupes of Big Pharma. This might seem a facile observation, but as N. Ann Davis has argued is common in cases of invisible disability, there is much insensitivity that results from the double bind requiring clarification. If you have an attack of senseless, dysfunctional pain, you can't say that it is entirely outside of yourself, nor are you planning a pride parade to claim it as your own. In fact, one musn't fight too much against the pain once an attack begins, as that only makes it much worse, as many child migraineurs can learn through relaxation therapy and biofeedback, because of all the muscular tension involved in bracing against pain.

So perhaps a logical way through the double bind is to recognize that imagining migraine as external, at risk of overlooking the solidarity of group identity or accepting victim-status, is actually a coping strategy and an important way of subjectively resisting trigemony. According to Eric Cassel,

> Suffering that occurs during acute illness seems to arise largely from sources external to the person – from injury or the disease. . . . When suffering occurs in the course of acute disease, medical understandings of the body and categories of disease seem adequate to explain why the threat to the integrity of the person exists. This is not so in chronic illness. . . . Suffering in chronic illness may also arise because the integrity of the person is threatened by internally

generated dissension between different aspects of the patient, despite the continuing perception that the threat is external.

(48–49)

Though primarily a method for depicting pain, externalization also provides a means of coping. Renée French says that *H Day* was inspired by a

> thing that I do to get through it [migraine] ... which is, um, visualizing a world. ... I used to lie down and try to not think about anything ... but now I kind of make up a world, so lying there, I have a wet washcloth on my forehead ... and I think about a place where there's no windows, no doors, just these buildings ... and then maybe a dog. It's enough that I start to forget about the pain a little bit ... not too stimulating.
>
> (Strand booktalk)

Migraine is such a narrowing, isolating experience that spatializing distraction or even eternalizing the imagined "source" of pain seems affirmative as an agentive response.

Migraineur's best friend

Imagining pain as contained and pushing it away from body, migraine art and comics depict action from outside the pain, disowning it. Like Kant ignoring his gout, such redirection is a coping distraction. But why does French imagine a dog in the process? The dog is a fixture of her migraine-scape:

> [P]art of dealing with my migraines is to imagine walking around in a place with giant blank buildings and enormous ships with nothing on them, and dogs. If I can concentrate on that place as purely as possible, I might fall asleep and wake up with at least a dent in the pain.
>
> (Comic Book Resources)

In French's fantasy landscape on the right-hand side, the migraineur's stand-in and ultimately the main character of the piece, who suffers but actively escapes the onslaught, is, significantly, man's best friend as pain proxy.

Speaking of the cover for *H Day* in her interview for *The Comics Reporter*, French told Tom Spurgeon that although "[y]ou could definitely pick a better drawing for the cover if you were going to explain what's inside the book," she picked it "because that was a breakthrough drawing for me. ... That dog is moving and that feels to me like a headache and when I made that drawing it was an 'a-ha' moment for me" (Spurgeon). Taking this comment as a cue, I reconsidered the cover (see figure 5.7)—does it not introduce keys to understanding the text? We see our hero, the dog, who has been lowered a package (that elsewhere resembles the folded washcloth so many migraineurs use for their forehead), and the dog's outlines are blurred. We know the dog is a "stand-in" for the migraineur

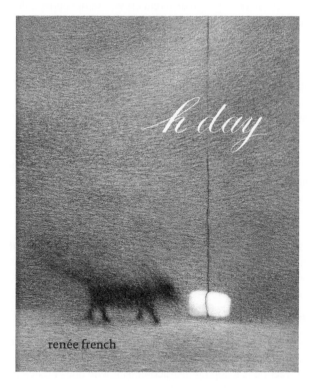

Figure 5.7 Renée French, *H Day*, 2010. Reprinted with permission of the artist.

from the left-hand panels—is he offered some relief from the towel? Or is he the pain itself here, who is becoming vaguely enveloped by the chance of relief in the same way that the left-hand side migraineur is enveloped through his senses by the bed he seeks refuge in? Is the blurring of pain a sign of hope? These possibilities make sense in the larger tradition of using animals in comics art and children's books.

Animals can create more empathy yet enable selective distancing more effectively than human figures. Michael Chaney calls animal proxies "approximate but affectless other(s)" and argues that "from vantages of dispassionate supervision, animals mark the space of witness" (130, 95). Suzanne Keen writes, in "Fast Tracks to Narrative Empathy: Anthropomorphism and Dehumanization in Graphic Narratives," that "[t]he artist's visual representation of animal faces and postures, featuring big eyes and upward-gazing attitudes of abjection, advantageously short-circuits readers' defensive distancing from dangerous predators that would usually invite antipathy" (142). Ideally, what results is a transferring of "sympathy of readers from the suffering fictional characters to real sufferers" (142). As Elaine Scarry has written of Miquel Angel Asturias's *Men of Maize*, in which a dog represents the pain of the protagonist, "Pain decontextualizes: it breaks the sufferer away from all other dimensions of his world, including his own body," expressing "the fact of pain and transferring it to another surface, the body of the dog" (2006, 30–31). The scene previously mentioned in my third chapter, from Bulgakov's *The Master and Margarita,* echoes this canine role in vicarious coping. Pontius Pilate's only relieving thoughts during his attack are of his dog, Banga, whom he wants to pet, complain to about his pain, and be comforted by (17–19). Pilate's fondness for his dog in turn makes him a more sympathetic character in the scene. When this externalization of internal pain onto an animal proxy[7] occurs, we can "stay" from and imagine the pain, or at least approach understanding its effect on the sufferer.

Cartoon violence is often thought of as desensitizing viewers to suffering, but it also models this coping power of projection. Animals can be even easier to project upon. Migraineur George Herriman made a career out of a seemingly simple plot line that would come to typify cartoon projection: Krazy Kat is in love with Ignatz the mouse, who in almost every strip hits Krazy in the head with a brick, which Krazy mistakes as a love token (see figure 5.8). Widely regarded as the most accomplished comics-strip artist in history, Herriman set the prototype for an endlessly repeatable storyline that would become a standard to Saturday morning cartoons as well. Ariela Freedman writes that "these anthropomorphized animals . . . and the repeated, mechanistic, sadomasochistic compulsion" allows the reader to be distant enough to "laugh at their pain" (383–384). The endlessly repeated pummeling of cartoon characters concretizes power in a currency children understand: pain and resilience.

The ever-present cartoon critters who repeatedly take on physical violence (and pop back to life) seem capable of vicariously taking on their creator's or audience's transferred pains, which is the theme of the most explicit pain proxy in comics—Grant Morrison's Coyote, Crafty. In no. 5 of *Animal Man,* is a metacomic episode,

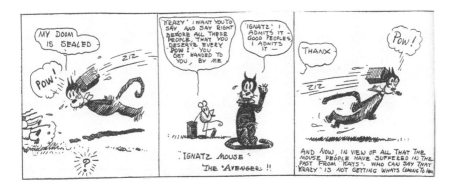

Figure 5.8 © George Herriman. 1920. Courtesy of Fantagraphics Books (fantagraphics.com)

"The Coyote Gospel," a coyote tale emphasizing the Promethean elements of its American Indian sources, in which Coyote, embodied in the cartoonish Crafty, resembles Wile E. Coyote. In a flashback setting deliberately stylized after television cartoons, Crafty revolts against the violence and cruelty of the fictive reality of the cartoon world: "No one in those days could remember a time when the world was free from strife . . . with bodies that renewed themselves instantly, following each wounding, no one thought to challenge the futile brutality of existence. Until Crafty."

Of course Crafty is punished by the gods for questioning, and suffers even more, as seen in a panel directly quoting the visual moment captured in so many paintings, including the Rubens piece (*Prometheus Bound*) many of the children chose in Scarry's "Among the School Children" as the best depiction of pain. We read that each wounding "taught new pain. Yet with each terrible death and resurrection, Crafty knew that by his torment, the world was redeemed." And in fact, the dog as pain proxy can work in such a cathartic, suffering, and redeeming way for the reader. The more widespread use of (usually domesticated) canines in children's film and TV might make it seem as if our culture simply heroically worships these animals, but in the comics of invisible suffering, their complicated fictional role as pain proxies also comes into sharper focus. Even Greg Fiering's Migraine Boy has a dog named "Tylenol" (see figure 5.9).

The pain proxy is both an imaginary projection and agent of interdependent resilience, at once a representative of the impaired person's subjectivity, the pain which threatens their ability to perceive clearly, and resistance to that pain. Like Scarry's "imagined agent" and Morrison's Crafty, French's pain proxy, the dog

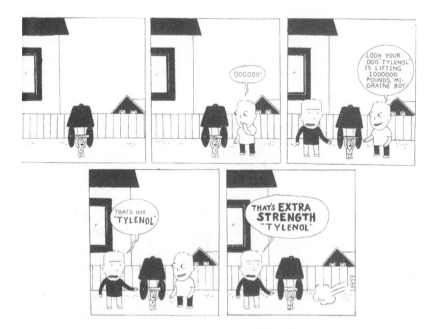

Figure 5.9 Greg Fiering, *Migraine Boy*, 2004. Reprinted with permission of the artist.

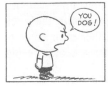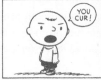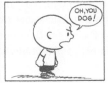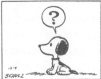

Figure 5.10 © Charles Schulz. 1952. Courtesy of Fantagraphics Books (fantagraphics.com).

hero, is able to serve as a stand-in for the human *and* human pain—a projection itself that is never politically neutral, as Donna Haraway warns: "[C]ontrary to lots of dangerous and unethical projection in the Western world that makes domestic canines into furry children, dogs are not about oneself" (11). This curious hierarchy seems to imply that dogs have more right to agency than children but is an effective reminder of the unchecked projection reflected on both. Dogs are especially seen in cultural productions as reflective of an impossible combination of unquestioning loyalty and responsibility, as Erica Fudge reminds, because we impose this construction on them: "[T]he pet's refusal to judge its owner is not, of course, a refusal, but a breakdown in communication. If a dog is judging its owner, how could we ever know?" (33). As an inherently silenced party, the pain proxy is infinitely reflexive: "The pet is a reassuring presence as it can never speak back, can never disagree, or if it does, can easily be punished" (33). The conflicts between disability- and animal-activism over the training and treatment of service dogs indicate how complicated this silence makes social definitions of rights-oriented justice (McHugh 228 n.3).

Dogs in comics occasionally take on our pain, and even allow us to love them and laugh at them at the same time—a kind of therapeutic sacrifice. If you consider the Peanuts strip from December 9, 1950, in which Charlie Brown dramatically berates Snoopy in language reminiscent of tragedy, you'll also note the comic nonchalance of the persevering beagle (see figure 5.10). Schulz highlights the somewhat ridiculous ways in which dogs serve as scapegoats and ideals of innocence at the same time. Beyond simply being sympathetic, animals in this dynamic culturally allow the detachment needed for the reader to "stay" just enough to remain other-oriented. And, they may serve as models for us to conceptualize agency in the face of trigemony.

Seeing rather than being pain

In 1882, Friedrich Nietzsche wrote,

> I have given a name to my pain and call it "dog." It is just as faithful, just as obtrusive and shameless, just as entertaining, just as clever as any other dog – and I can scold it and vent my bad mood on it, as others do with their dogs, servants, and wives.
>
> (249–250)

To quickly move beyond Nietzsche's offensive hierarchy of abuse, I prefer to focus on his identification of pain with a loyal and abusable pet, a canine representation of his invisible discomfort. Nietzsche's dog-called-pain brings a particularly relevant insight to this process for the migraineur, providing further explanation of the pain proxy not simply as potentially abusive, but as an expression of resilience in the face of pain.

In *Thus Spoke Zarathustra*, Nietzsche compares the human ego with animals' (cited in Acampora 55). Debra B. Bergoffen explains that Nietzsche

> contrasts a "cat-egotism" with a "dog-egotism." More recently domesticated than dogs, cats were never herd animals and have never regarded humans as "masters." So much the better, says Nietzsche, as he disparages the dog as "that lazy, tail-wagging parasite which has become 'dog-like' only through being the slave of man."
>
> (Acampora 252)

One can assume, then, that his equating of pain with a being he views as so debased is a desperate declaration of domination. Critics often reduce Nietzsche's "dog" to representing anything from ennui to angst, but few give the most obvious and straightforward reading much shrift. Nietzsche, as a migraineur and with later illness as well, struggled intensely and frequently with pain—real pain that's not necessary to metaphorically mask to understand. His proclamation is one of trying to master his pain, and he is both angry and amused (all the more interesting if you consider this in the light of his heavy use of opium at the time of this writing). In "Dogs, Domestication, and the Ego," Gary Shapiro argues,

> How liberating it would be if we could see our "pain" – the sum of our resentments and frustrations, for example – as a dog that frequently amuses us but needs to be kept in its place and can serve as an outlet for our bad temper. This would be far superior to seeing ourselves as identical with the pain, and the same holds true for our relation to the ego, which follows us about like a dog.
>
> (Acampora, 55)

More importantly, I think, Kathleen Marie Higgins pegs it: "[By seeing one's pain as a dog, one can take attitudes toward it, and not simply *be* it" (108). Fictional animal proxies allow us to imagine projecting pain as a way of disclaiming that pain as our own. Migraine has no wound to show, no weapon to blame, and no swarming attack to flee. But in providing proxies, migraine art and comics allow us to vicariously master pain, imagining an escape. They allow us to have an attitude toward pain rather than simply being it.

This is not to suggest that work like that of George Herriman and Renée French encourages an abusive view. It does help to suggest, however, the elaborate functionality of comics' canines or any pain proxy, especially in the challenging cases in which they reflect human suffering that is otherwise invisible, perhaps even otherwise unbearable. In a similar process, Jennette Fulda imagines yoking her head pain in a similar manner: "Instead of living *in* pain, perhaps I could learn to live *with* pain, as if it were my partner instead of my master" (211). Likewise, such animal proxies can demonstrate imaginative coping through externalizing or transferring pain and caring about the pain of others, effecting through visualization the mastering, or at least living with, migraine.

Migraine is liminal in terms of medical understanding, despite the fact that it most certainly has existed as long as humans have: "The pathophysiology of migraine is complex, and over 20 years of exhaustive research [since advancements in understanding pain mechanisms] has failed to unravel the mystery of this common malady" (Chakravarty and Sen 228). We now know, at least, that migraine is trigeminovascular—both a vascular (creating nociceptive pain) and neural (ultimately neuropathic, caused by central and peripheral hypersensitization) experience. It is sometimes an isolated (acute) incident, more often episodic, and sometimes becomes chronic. On one hand it can be held up theoretically as challenging binaries that have been abandoned by pain specialists since the mid-1980s but are still dominant paradigms in the public imagination: physical/emotional, "real"/psychosomatic, and visible/invisible. But ontologically, though it may seem to fall back on Cartesian mind/body dualism to say so, the projection of pain as "not me" is a necessary splitting in validating migraineurs' identity as separate from their pain in spite of it. We must accept that pain is part of the migraine experience, but we can reject dysfunctional pain as a part of our identity even as it impairs us. And like Nietzsche, George Herriman, and Renée French, if we channel our autonomous will into an imaginary vessel, we are not denying but reaffirming our agency.

If like Bob Flanagan, we can have a sense of humor about it, even better. In *Sick: The Life and Death of Bob Flanagan, Supermasochist*, Flanagan displays one of his pieces titled "Visible Man," which is basically a plastic medical model of a human being with internal organs visible—but he has fabricated realistic bodily fluids, which ooze from all orifices. Petra Kuppers describes the importance of such visibility, as it helps us to ask these questions: "Who inflicts pain here? Is there a distinction between body and self? Is Flanagan at somebody's mercy, or somebody's pity?" (82). And these questions have probably always surrounded persons with dysfunctional pain. In 1967, Abby Adams described a similar project enacted at the prompting of a child migraineur during play therapy: "One patient, a ten-year old boy, had openly expressed a desire to put together a Visible Head," which he used to project his experience (and perhaps imagine, like Nietzsche and his hypothetical dog, vicariously imposing his pain on another)—"[H]e described a repetitive nightmare . . . [which] involved the insertion into the brain of a 'long, black pin' which was small when it first was put in and expanded after insertion. . . . He fantasied the needle being inserted frontally, which was the locus of his headaches" (139). The psychoanalyst predictably interprets this symbolism sexually, but there is a more straightforward level on which the Visible Head helps a patient express, conceptually get outside of, and imagine controlling "what actually goes on inside his skull" (138). This is an empowering performance of vicariously counterattacking pain. The consistency with which child migraineurs analogize the attacks with violent weapons from an outside force indicates they are also already asking the same questions Flanagan's work asks, and therapeutic play with the Visible Head allows the boy to symbolically imagine controlling migraine—seeing the head rather than being trapped in its pain.

Notes

1 Ian Williams has coined the term "graphic medicine" for this growing subgenre.
2 Green's protagonist (self) asks, looking in the mirror, "How can they know I'm struggling if I don't look sick?" (212). She even uses a coping mechanism similar to that I describe in chapter 3, "Slowly, I learned to disconnect from the chatter in my head . . . and from the expanding sensations in my body. I could choose to separate myself" (192).
3 In her analysis of advertisements for pain remedies, comparing and contrasting ads in publications for doctors with those for general readership, Scarry concludes that pain-reliever ads "that make their way into the wide public realm represent both the pain and the cessation of pain only as they can be perceived from the outside" (1994, 25). Because everyone experiences pain, customers don't require reminding of that, but the appeal to outer observable consequences remind why "it must be gotten rid of" (1994, 26).
4 G.D. Schott tweaks this idea in a useful manner: "[T]he same difficulties in expression arise for those experiencing other unpleasant sensory and emotional states – for example the schizophrenic who attempts to describe his auditory hallucinations, or the epileptic his olfactory aura. Rather, pain is intrinsically impossible to convey to others, and there-fore language will always prove inadequate. The same inadequacy arises for the blind person who tries to express what he 'sees'" (209). Scarry is a language-centered scholar who is reflecting not only her disciplinary bias and medium, but her cultural bias as well. Wolf et al. argue "Anglo-Americans see pain as information about the individual's body, whereas Italians see pain as a disruption of interpersonal life" (148 n. 2).
5 Katalin Orbán writes, "[V]ision is a powerful regime of abstraction that presupposes distance and is a rival form of world-making" (58).
6 Though many sources on hemispheric dominance (left-brain versus right-brain) oversim-plify it, because migraine is typically a unilateral experience, it is worth addressing. Psy-chologist Stanley Coren has popularized the perception that migraine is twice as likely in left-handed children, which seems to have taken purchase in some practices (194). Southpaw journalist Melissa Roth recounts her first visit to a neurologist in the 1990s: "The first question he asked, before I could tell him about my migraine headaches, was 'Are you left-handed?'" (12). Just for the record, two of the most popular left-handers to be proudly claimed in histories of left-handedness are, quite relevantly here, Friedrich Nietzsche and Lewis Carroll.
  A 2002 study tested the hypothesis that "unilateral headache sufferers might experi-ence pain in their hand-dominant hemisphere" but found "no correlation between the side the unilateral head pain manifests itself on and the dominant hand" (Lipscombe and Prior, 146, 148). But some of us are not dominant in the hemisphere that our handedness would suggest, or have "bilateral" (non)dominance. One 1987 study concluded, more specifically, that "[s]tudents who identified themselves as ambidextrous were at approxi-mately 50% greater risk than right-handers and left-handers of experiencing headaches," proposing that "If unilateral cerebral information overload provokes migrainous episodes and nondominant hemispheres have low overload thresholds, then ambidextrous people would be at increased risk of headaches because they are more likely than others to have two nondominant hemispheres" (Kilty et al. 159, 162). This hypothesis merits further consideration (or debunking), especially if popular oversimplification of "left-brain" and "right-brain" children persists.

7 This belief is not just demonstrated in fiction but also in historic treatments. These, however, can be less sympathetic acts of transference. Consider this passage from Frazer's
Golden Bough describing a practice from the ninth century: "When a Moor has a headache he will sometimes take a lamb or a goat and beat it till it falls down, believing that
the headache will thus be transferred to the animal" (vol. 9, 31). In an example relevant
to migraine in particular, eighteenth-century physician David Hartley wrote of the coun-
terirritating emetic effects of opiates, which "abate much, soon after the Narcotic is
ejected by Vomiting; also because whipping a Dog, after he has taken the *Nux Vomica*,
contributes to obviate its ill effects" (51). *Nux Vomica* was prescribed for epilepsy and
migraine at the time. Emily Dickinson, for example, had a prescription for it; it is still
used homeopathically. See Lyndall Gordon (216). For a discussion of Emily Dickinson as
migraineur, see Andrew Levy. The dog seems to commonly serve as a pain proxy in common figures of speech as well. The prescription of beating a dog also echoes the concept
of counterirritation introduced by Martin Pernick in my second chapter, as does, simply,
the idea of taking "the hair of the dog that bit you." Pain proxies in comics are similarly externalized receptors and expressions of intersubjectively invisible experience.
Beyond metaphor, their visual complexity allows endless, even contradictory, projection
rather than ideological shorthand. For an unusual diagnosis of cluster headache in two
eighteenth-century servants who'd tended a rabid dog and her litter, see Eadie (200–201).

Conclusion
Animality, empathy, and interdependence

Like children, whose pain control was considered of lesser medical importance until the late 1980s in the United States (Bridgeman 2002, Webb 2004), nonhuman animals have been palliatively redefined throughout history for the convenience of adult humans. According to Descartes,

> If an animal is a mere automaton made by the hand of God . . . then it cannot experience pain. . . . The yelp of a dog is not an expression of pain, it is merely a mechanical response to an external stimuli, on par with the relationship between a clock and its alarm.
>
> (quoted in Fudge 98–99)

Where it befits human adult interests, silenced subjects can be miscast as in or out of pain to suit nefarious ends.[1]

Both disability and childhood have been historically defined by oppressive discourses that dehumanize through comparisons with animals. Susan McHugh argues, in *Animal Stories: Narrating across Species Lines*, that such dehumanizing plays a pivotal role in reifying speciesist, ableist, and I would add ageist, norms:

> I do not want to downplay the damage done by the historically stigmatizing association of disabled and other people with animals, but rather to pinpoint how the humanist subject becomes produced through these connections. Often they are forged within the extremely volatile medical and biological discourses in which animal proximities threaten the so-called normal human subject with metaphorical no less than bodily harm, even as they become means of representing the experience of being human.
>
> (31)

Allegiance with impaired persons, with children, and with nonhuman animals all require a decentering of certain norms which impede empathy for and recognition of silenced needs. But in the case of nonverbal adults, prearticulate young, and nonhumans we still have to largely rely upon (sometimes imperfect or retrospective) representations projected to bridge understanding. The figure of the runt can embody the intersection of such experience in discourse.

Though nonhuman animals, like children, are objects for endless cultural projection, they are also shown as bridges to empathy and connection, especially in the vulnerable, potentially cast-off but ultimately resilient figures of surviving runts. Niall Griffiths demonstrates such a position with optimistic empowerment in his novel *Runt* (2007). The teenaged narrator of *Runt* is living with epilepsy, calling his seizures "My Times" and describing them and the natural world in a style that recalls mystic Opal Whiteley: "I liked very much knowing every raindrop by name and liked it too that the owl and the lady fox and every last bit of rain knew my name back as well" (29). He is particularly responsive to the youngest and most vulnerable members of animal families, as demonstrated with his bond to the runt of the farm cat Charlesworth's litter: "The other kittens didn't bite but *this* one did even tho it was the smallest cos it had been chosen to be the one that bit" (31–32). When he sees a nest of harrier chicks he wonders, "[I]f birds like that had babies like Charlesworth . . . their babies would be different to the others, a different colour and a different size and a different Way in it to the others in the nest with him. I hoped they did" (48). It is through this young character's imagination that we see modeled not only empathy for vulnerability during precarious infancy, but also difference and resilience celebrated. Literary childhoods abound with such interspecies compassion.

The connection between empathy for nonhuman animals and empathy for children is deeply historical. That the development of U.S. child rights laws *followed* those defending animal rights should be a concrete reminder of this link—the first child abuse case in the United States in defense of Mary Ellen Wilson having been brought forward in 1874 by the American Society for the Prevention of Cruelty to Animals. Lewis Carroll, the figure so central to both children's literature and migraine writing, was also an early animal-rights proponent who wrote that "the prevention of suffering to a human being does not justify the infliction of a greater amount of suffering on an animal" (quoted in Jaques, 44). For Carroll, clearly the same compassionate and emancipatory views toward childhood were easily applicable to nonhuman animals. And as Susan E. Lederer discusses, in the twentieth-century United States, "Children received most of the attention of animal protectionists" (102). Like Descartes and his dog, many medical experimenters have used their own children as experimental subjects, and "like dogs and cats, infants and orphans were unable to protect themselves from ambitious investigators" (101). The twentieth-century shift toward greater protection of children posed a slippery slope in the minds of animal-rights activists. In the 1930s, the Vivisection Investigation League even protested the emerging protectionism prioritizing children over nonhuman animals in a pamphlet arguing, "It is not a question of Your Dog or Your Baby, but one of Your Dog AND Your Baby. It is NOT a question of animals or human beings, but one of animals AND human beings" (Lederer 101). Whether one is willing to recognize similar protections for nonhuman animals, the tradition of recognizing child pain is linked to this longer tradition of debating animal pain. And, ironically, because veterinarians today receive far more training in pain care than other doctors (with nonverbal patients, no less), according to Christine Chambers, "your dog could get better pain care than you or your child."

Less controversially and more universally linked is the compassion of children for animals with potential compassion for the pain of other children. Michael Chaney writes of an

> axiom of children's literature, in which animal representations echo earlier traditions of the fable, myth, and fairy tale. One effect of this harkening back to primitive culture is that the device of animal representation becomes in itself a signifier for children . . . occupying a proximate position to the animal as well.
>
> (132–133)

Certainly this principle is evident in *My Seizure Dog*, with words and pictures by Evan Moss (seven years old at time of publication)—service dogs and therapy dogs are represented as proxies for impaired experience. Moss imagines that his seizure dog will "go everywhere with me" and be his "best friend." Lori Jo Oswald adds that a common humanizing message of children's literature is, ironically, to identify closely with nonhuman animals:

> [P]art of the child's "growing up" is due to his or her standing up to a person who is cruel to an animal. . . . The child knows that the mistreatment of an animal is wrong, and no matter what the consequences, he or she must act to rescue the animal victim.
>
> (145)

Such moments reflect a larger tradition in which readers learn both compassion and humane action as regards an oppressed other whose pain may move us but also remains silently contained.

Books and films representing children as living with impairment through empowered alternative ability are still not plentiful in every classroom for a general audience: "Many professionals indicated they would include literature about a disability only when a child with a disability became a member of that class" (Blaska 1). This dearth of diverse representation does not prepare children, and the adults they become, to understand invisible impairments like dysfunctional pain when they will encounter them in others or themselves. And whereas the politics of disability have fostered movements unifying and empowering impaired individuals through supportive group identity and activism, Elizabeth Wheeler has pointed out a distinct challenge in creating disability solidarity among impaired children, who are (temporally) limited by necessary dependence upon adults to first help them to access others with shared experience and discover the power of community:

> Disability studies emphasizes the public profile of disability as a shared culture, a community, and a political movement. A core value of the discipline is

the social model of disability, as opposed to the individual model. However, most children don't grow up around others who share their disability.

(Wheeler 335)

Of course, Internet groups may suggest an outlet, but these are compromised, as Kuppers and Marko have pointed out, by potentially undetectable but exploitative pharmaceutical bias, and opportunities for community-building are fewer for children, whose socializing might not transcend the family or school. Empathy must be exercised in social and institutional practice, through flexibility in school policy and structure with further medical testing, which depend upon adult advocacy. Cindy Dell Clark writes, "Adults easily miss the degree to which children's lives are encumbered by dependency and control. . . . Child powerlessness is doubly the case for chronically ill children" (145). Children are marginalized subjects in our culture; so are persons with invisible disability:

> [Y]oung . . . people with chronic illnesses inhabit a category not easily understood or accepted. We are considered too young to be ill for the rest of our lives, yet we are not expecting cure or recovery. We cannot be granted the time-out that is normally granted to the acutely ill (or if we were given it at first and now used it up, overused it), yet we seem to refuse to return to a pre-illness life. We are not old enough to have finished making our contributions of productivity.
>
> (Wendell 21)

And so our alternate needs for ability must be recognized and respected. Representing these experiences to children (with dignity and promoting empathy) is even more necessary for children to develop solidarity.

Animal proxies, at least, are ubiquitous in children's books and movies in classrooms and homes. And they can instruct against the cultural denial of our shared bodily vulnerabilities by encouraging interdependence in its place. The most relevant example to my argument, among the classics found in most school libraries and many homes, is E. B. White's *Charlotte's Web* (1952), which taps some of the deepest, most difficult issues of feeling cast out, burdensome, and threatened by perceived "weakness." In it Fern Arable and her father have this fraught discussion over his plans to kill the runt of a pig litter:

> "Fern," said Mr. Arable, "I know more about raising a litter of pigs than you do. A weakling makes trouble. Now run along!"
>
> "But it's unfair," cried Fern. "The pig couldn't help being born small, could it? If *I* had been very small at birth, would you have killed *me*?"
>
> (3)

Fern has asked the unspeakable question by projecting on an animal proxy. It is a question children are perceptive enough to ponder. Whether the vulnerable newborn shall survive a precarious infancy has been well-debated within ethics and disability politics[2]—most eloquently, perhaps, by Harriet McBryde Johnson (2003). I have taken up instead the matter of how we can recognize and support the thriving of the small or disadvantaged members who survive into a sometimes still precarious childhood, especially when those in need have been silenced and over-looked because their impairment is invisible or leads to their being dismissed as wimps, whiners, and fakers. This territory in childhood has been less explored than more sensational conflicts, as Cindy Dell Clark has redressed by asking, "[W]hat about the child who carries a lasting, medically treatable chronic condition, an ill-ness a child must learn to live with rather than die from? This child, of course, also deserves attention and compassion" (2). One of the most common complaints of children who live with invisible disabilities, chronic illness, or fluctuating impair-ment is the perception others project upon them of burdensome weakness, which results in feeling cast out yet more dependent upon others for care.

Fern Arable learns that only through intervention do certain beings live, and with that intervention comes a commitment to aid their survival until it is more certain. Runts in the wild are often abandoned; runts in "civilization" require spe-cial attention. Periodically, I have used references to our common animality as a way of making both scapegoating and interdependence explicit. In her YA novel, *Accidents of Nature* (2006), Harriet McBryde Johnson does this with brutal beauty, imagining first the natural setting for her novel, a camp for children living with varied impairments, built on the edge of a wild forest of trees, each of which rep-resents the overlooked diversity of human bodies as well:

> At this stage, no amount of management could change their basic nature. Thin and thick, twisted and shapely, bent and straight, they remained. Unrehabili-tated. They were products of what is called the natural law of survival of the fittest. But their fitness was not defined by human needs, or market forces, or any grand design. In truth, they did not survive because they were fit. Rather, they were proven fit because they survived. They survived by accident.
>
> (2–3)

In the midst of such a naturalistic view, the narrator of *Accidents of Nature*, Jean, a teenager with cerebral palsy, awakens to a freshly politicized awareness tinged by the angst of her indebtedness: "It is my family's love that saved me as a baby and has carried me safe thus far" (223). This debt can be an emotional burden to chil-dren growing up within a culture that insists upon denying human vulnerability. We are all accidents of nature, but survival also depends upon culture, especially for children born with life-threatening or chronic impairments.

Some of us know this dependence all too well, as adults who survived a precari-ous childhood. We know the vulnerability of our animal bodies, and if we are lucky enough to survive and be cared for and thrive with the support of the social body, the experience makes us empathetic. In *Bodies in Revolt*, Ruth O'Brien argues that animality can equalize us in interdependence: "Our bodies could unite us, creat-ing a very expansive concept if the myth of independence is abandoned" (115). Recent developments in the anti-vaccination movement demonstrate the dangers of parents thinking about health as a personal or family issue rather than a shared community responsibility, and citizens cannot see how completely ignored children's individual rights to health are when we conflate their interests with parental rights. Eula Biss writes, "Herd immunity, an observable phenomenon, now seems implausible only if we think of our bodies as inherently disconnected from other bodies. Which, of course, we do" (2014, 20). And, of course, her implication is that we should not. Recognizing our corporeal animal vulnerability and cultural interdependence for health are necessary steps toward well-being for all (interconnected) bodyminds. Most of us will be impaired at some point in our lives. Disability activists and advocates show us that when we accept our vulnerabilities as well as our responsibilities to care for each other, we might begin to undo the damage of socially imposed disability, and we will thrive all the better by acknowledging the unique abilities of our fellow runts.

There is a good reason children identify easily with animals, especially runts, as smaller, disadvantaged, or even cast-away offspring. Like nonhuman animals who live in a human-dominated world, children are particularly vulnerable, powerless, and potentially dependent upon others for survival. When Fern Arable rescues the runt pig Wilbur in E. B. White's *Charlotte's Web*, she recognizes his shared animal vulnerability, and his need for protection. She also commits in that moment to serving as proxy for his voice, and to advocacy toward another's survival and well-being.

Unlike some fellow creatures, humans are not born able to fend for ourselves. Our prolonged gestation and dependence mean that our culture must reinforce nurturing. In her chapter, "How to Save Your Life: Lessons from a Runt Pig," Karen Coats writes that "all humans (and some pigs) are born prematurely, and [Fern] understands that it is the task of someone else to save their lives" (15). Fern, and later the spider Charlotte, will save Wilbur "by speaking for him, by connecting him to the world of language" (16). In this book I use the term "runt" to truthfully acknowledge our animalistic reality—runts can be spurned, by community, family, sometimes even parents. Some overcome the vulnerable years and are labeled survivors, others "wimps," but all should be recognized as thriving individuals with a right to autonomy and their own unique agency. Embracing runthood as tough and thriving also blunts the marginalizing force of the label's traditional usage but presses us to nonetheless recognize vulnerabilities we all have in common to varying degrees, instead celebrating a potential solidarity with each other and children who experience debilitating, stigmatized, or chronic impairment. Words might not heal, but they can help us to recognize, unify, and support each other when such perspectives are silenced or invisible. Disability politics can inform us with a democratic zeal that serves everyone. But for children, who are less likely to organize because their public sphere is more limited to family or school, solidarity requires a degree of adult advocacy. Those born or living with impairments that require medical intervention, public accommodation, empathy, and dignified treatment, must be recognized as a unique political interest but shared investment. Regardless of what impairs us individually, we must reach a consensual awareness, advocating for each other and our younger counterparts.

As mammals, we are equipped with a capacity for pain as a warning system—but that system can go awry, resulting in misunderstood dysfunctional pain syndromes. Nature also equips mammals with a lesser-known capacity for forgetting pain once resolved—a capacity that can make adults less empathetic with child pain that has no visible source. Forgetting pain unfortunately makes it easier to ignore in others. But our bodies carry these memories even as we adapt, grow, and become more powerful members of the social body. We must use that power to help others in pain, and in order to fully empathize, we need to remember, not simply "protect."

Protectionism can result in a less visible form of oppression, like the regulatory history of the twentieth and twenty-first centuries, wherein pain patients suffer more than the prescription abusers and illegal sales such regulations are meant to stop. In the cases of children, advocacy is a precarious business—protection rights must be balanced with equal opportunities for participation, even self-determination. Children deserve more than protection—they should also have opportunities for therapy that equal those of adults (and in fact, in CRC-ratifying countries,[3] this too is at least legally recognized as a birthright, if not always in practice). However, as a legacy to the cultural denial of child pain, the emphasis on protection over participation has resulted in children with many conditions being therapeutic orphans. Kept "safe" from serving as subjects in medical trials, children have fewer treatment options and often depend upon chance off-label prescriptions, which are particularly common in use for migraine (Loder 636). Even worse, when combined with social forces like the punitively focused war on drugs, less harmful therapies remain inaccessible due to criminalization. For a recent and highly relevant example, consider the plight of "marijuana refugees."

By now numbering in the thousands, parents have become activists in the interest of legally developing cannabis treatments for children, and many have moved to Colorado for access to cannabidiol in particular for their children with seizure disorders (Schwartz 2015). In 2012, at the behest of the parents of Charlotte Figi, then a five-year-old with a rare form of life-threatening epilepsy called Dravet syndrome that resulted in "sometimes hundreds of seizures in a day," grower Josh Stanley and his brothers developed a cannabis oil that reduced Charlotte's seizures to just one in her first week of treatment (Schwartz). If cannabidiol can do that for severe and life-threatening impairments, imagine what it could do for children with migraine, for which the dominant prophylactic treatments are the same anticonvulsants used for seizures, with many unwanted side effects.

According to Ethan Russo, "Cannabis, or marijuana, has been used for both symptomatic and prophylactic treatment of migraine. It was highly esteemed as a headache remedy by the most prominent physicians of the age between 1874 and 1942," including nineteenth-century neurologist of literary infamy, Silas Weir Mitchell and Dr. William Osler, who recommended *Cannabis indica* "the most satisfactory remedy" for migraine as late as 1913 (1, 4). In 1891 physician J. B. Mattison advocated that "the most important use of cannabis was in treating 'that opprobrium of the healing art—migraine'" (cited in Grinspoon 6–7). The Stanley brothers, who created Charlotte's oil, include migraine, PTSD, cancer, and heart disease among the conditions it can be used to treat. They call their pediatric tincture, perhaps with full poetic awareness, Charlotte's Web. In March of 2015 a bipartisan bill was introduced calling for nonpsychoactive cannabis products like cannabidiol, which do not contain THC, to be declassified as Schedule 1 substances. Though unlikely to receive adequate support, the Charlotte's Web Medical Access Act (H.R. 1635) could bring untold numbers of therapeutic orphans into fuller control of their own lives and daily well-being.

The discourse surrounding the case of Charlotte Figi, including a *Dateline* episode and Ted Talk by Josh Stanley, is not free of curist rhetoric like "these children get their lives back" or "parents get their children back," and Charlotte is sometimes invoked in the poster-child tradition as a "courageous little girl." But there is little doubt that this less risky treatment actually saves lives and makes others more livable. In spite of the imperfect discourse, such moments succeed at bringing greater visibility to therapeutic orphans and at least promise to reeducate American adults about chronic illness, impairment, and children's rights to equal access in their efforts toward self-determination, health, and well-being.

If children with chronic illness or impairment are not granted a voice, we have to learn new dimensions of listening—reading between stoic lines. Voicing projects of childhood studies are a step in the right direction. But, as demonstrated by the visibility activism of queer and disability politics, sometimes words are simply not enough. In *Charlotte's Web*, when the voiceless animals rally to save the runt pig Wilbur, they not only use words, but they succeed because of interdependent solidarity and Charlotte's sacrificial visual display. She weaves words into her spectacular web, demonstrating the power of visibility to jolt viewers into a more empathetic perspective. In a less spectacular but nonetheless fascinating manner, the compulsory narratives demanded from persons with invisible impairments, and the visibility projects used to express, document, and legitimize their experiences, can be utilized together to materialize and make trivialized conditions like migraine, and the children living with it, more socially visible.

Notes

1 According to Melanie Joy, he brutally tried to prove his point: "Descartes nailed the paws of his wife's dog to a board in order to dissect it alive and prove that, unlike humans but like other animals, the dog was a soulless 'machine' whose cries of pain were no different from the springs and wheels of a clock automatically reacting when dismantled" (109).
2 For the dark side of these debates, see Kuhse and Singer. For an example of how personal voicing can counter disabling rhetoric, read Harriet McBryde Johnson (2003).
3 The Convention on the Rights of the Child "explicitly references children with disabilities. It is the first human rights treaty to include disability within its stipulated prohibited grounds of discrimination (Article 2), as well as to dedicate an entire article to children with disabilities. Article 23 calls upon states to 'recognize that a mentally or physically disabled child should enjoy a full and decent life, in conditions which ensure dignity, promote self-reliance and facilitate the child's active participation in the community'" (Sabatello 465–66).

Afterword

Scars (a migraine diary)

Somewhere deep beneath her fearless risk-taking, passive manipulation, and fierce show-stopping contralto, my mother has hidden any resentment for my almost killing her—and almost dying too.

I almost killed her twice. First, in a difficult birth requiring interventions, from which she hemorrhaged, a clot penetrated the heart and blood filled her lungs. The second time I was the distraction from her seeing an oncoming van running a stop sign, before she could brake in time. The bruise on her chest from our VW station wagon's steering wheel set off another clot. Again with her heart and lungs filling red.

But there were also the crises my own vulnerabilities forced upon the family. I was quite clearly the runt of the litter. From the beginning, my story (at least from the perspective of the litter) has been tied up with medical intervention. When it was time for my birth I was twisted in a brow position so that the umbilical cord wrapped around my neck. All that my mother heard was a slap and silence. She would not see me until later in an incubator. I wasn't premature, just a little puny and fairly maladapted—and have been ever since. Perhaps that is why the identity I felt my family reflected for me has always seemed connected to medical stories. My body and chance gave us plenty of events to hang narratives around.

At age three I became toxic (later we would learn, from chronic kidney infections, caused by a common malformation of the right ureter). I was too young to articulate what I was physically feeling and was eventually paralyzed into speechlessness anyway, but my body was so full of scar tissue that my organs weren't floating. Encephalitis set in, and I had to be hospitalized, but the doctor seemed uncertain about the cause, refusing to treat my symptoms lest that "mask" the root problem. After two weeks of total paralysis, dramatic weight loss, and undertreated fever, my case looked hopeless, so the doctor told my parents to prepare for my death—but with seemingly nothing left to lose, they snuck in a second opinion from a younger specialist who immediately suspected a constricted ureter (something easily treatable today with laser surgery). And after emergency exploratory surgery, for which I was quickly (and with some dramatic music, I imagine) cut open from spine to navel—scar tissue removed, given a renal abscess—the doctor upgraded the prognosis a bit: I might live, but I'd be brain damaged and require frequent dialysis.

My body refused to follow that fate, exercising the tiny resistance and free will sometimes allowed wee mites in the medical world. I got lucky. Instead of brain damage I got a smallish frame and mere migraine. Or perhaps that's only a coincidence—after all, doctors agree that the condition is usually hereditary. And my mother and maternal grandfather *were* migraineurs of a sort. But there must be some reason why I'd had as many attacks as they both had in their entire lives combined by the time I was five or six years old, and those attacks were only a shade of what would come a few years later. My condition would become severe, and in some periods of my life, almost chronically debilitating. Even though I barely remember anything about my hospitalized month in 1970, I am convinced that the protracted brain fever and undertreated pain complicated my neurological health, and that I will never shed the influence of those experiences, or the body that bears their traces.

Still my stories are not really my own. This was made especially clear to me in my early forties, when I spent much of a sabbatical in my hometown. Even then some people I ran into who'd known my parents when I was younger would first utter, "I remember when you were *so* sick . . ." Needless to say, I barely remember those events from almost half a century before, but this comment echoed the most common greeting (I kid you not, the *exact* words) I heard throughout my childhood from adults who seemed to marvel, a bit rudely, I thought, that I wasn't dead. My mother's border Munchausen's and my own budding hypochondria aside, such remarks affected me profoundly. I came to see myself as a medical burden—both survivor and weakling, an impression that would be reinforced as I grew into a life of embarrassingly lousy excuse-making, "Sorry I can't stay and play, I have a headache." There's probably not a migraineur alive who doesn't rue how weak that sounds.

The most profound result of being a child with severe and frequent migraine is not simply exposure to extraordinary discomfort, helplessness, and pain—it is the shock of alienation in discovering that others don't have this hidden yoke, bearing down at the least convenient times and robbing their dignity, leaving desperate pleas for help unanswerable, forcing us to realize that even our parents can't help us, and finally wondering that if *normal* people don't have this: what am I doing *wrong*?

But even worse, for me, was my dawning suspicion of an unspoken answer to the secretly nagging question, "*Can people really love something—someone—that nature has spurned?*"

When I was a teenager my family's basset hound, Meg, gave birth to a litter of five healthy puppies. But to the side, under a blanket we found a sixth abandoned with her birth sac on, suffocating her breaths, which formed bubbles around her mouth. My mother heroically grabbed her up, tore the sac, and wiped the puppy down. She didn't even have to think. But our dog's, Meg's, instinct had been different. The mother knows?

I can still remember the names for each of those puppies except one. Yes, that dappled little red-and-white runt. After such a dramatic entrance, she may not have even got one.

Red

The color children most associate with pain is red.[1] According to Alexander Theroux, "It is the first color of the newly born and the last seen on the deathbed" (159). My reflections on a migrainous childhood are full of red. My name was embroidered in red on the Snoopy towel I used as a nap mat in kindergarten, but I never could sleep because naptime came after a sugar-filled snack (a double-whammy trigger). An ever-pervasive ingredient at kiddy events in the 1970s was Kool-Aid—why anyone ever considered dye[2] and sugar water kid-friendly is beyond me. Red (why pretend they are actual fruit flavors?) was the favorite kind—and an automatic trigger for attacks. My body learned by age five not to drink it. Even the thought of it now floods my tongue with bile.

One year in elementary school dry Jell-O was a hot commodity. You'd wet your finger, dip it in the packet, and suck off the powder, also red (no child with any sense of lunchroom trade-value would dream of bringing lime or lemon flavors). It turned your finger bright pink. Needless to say, that wasn't good for migraine either. One month pomegranates were the rage. I loved the garnet gem-like seeds and the fact that this was a snack that didn't make me sick. But they weren't seasonal for long.

On the playground, red was the color that seeped through my eyelids when I tried to shut out the sun's stabbing light. It was the color of the blood throbbing over my temple into the tender territory just above and behind my eyebrow. It was also the color of those old rubber kickballs (which I feared would hit my head and trigger an attack).

I once witnessed my father mercifully killing a mouse in our backyard that our cat had been torturing loudly but only fatally wounding. He was brave enough to put the mouse "out of his pain" with a brick. Perhaps that scene was the inspiration for my asking him to knock me unconscious when I had a bad migraine, which he most likely thought was my being overdramatic, but in fact, it was something I thought about obsessively: if someone took a good swing with a thick board and hit the offending part of my body just so, couldn't they just knock me unconscious? Wouldn't that be, at least temporarily, a relief? Anybody who has to ask, "But wouldn't your head hurt more when you came to?" has never had severe migraine, or they would know that in fact a common distraction migraineurs create from the pain is another pain—perhaps a more sensible, controllable, cool-blue pain to counterbalance the red-hot hurt.

In fourth grade, I was labeled a remedial reader and taken out of the classroom every week for a forced speed-reading therapy session, which consisted of being set in front of an electronic screen that scrolled through a reading, one line lit at a time at a controlled pace—a machine teaching me not to linger on the language or even comprehend what I mechanically sounded out in my head, as if words mattered only in number, not meaning. The headaches became uncontrollable. Every Monday afternoon I would face the pea-green wall of the nurse's office where I would lie on a cot behind a pulled curtain and wait for my mother to pick me up, knowing that until I managed to sleep, the pain would continue to worsen. I just had to close my eyes and wait.

Luckily I was able to move to an alternative school the next school year where tracking wouldn't kill all the joys of learning. No more electronically enforced "speed reading" to catch up to a conformist standard of grade-level reading. No more Monday afternoons left alone in a room, staring at a dehumanizing screen, followed by that sad green wall.

Red is the color of pain's yoke, which lays bare the lie of free will. If one imagines pain as a glowing ember whose heat and intensity of light increases at the slightest sound or movement, threatening to grow to an inexpressible, self-destroying magnitude, then that glowing is the thing I focus on dimming through quiet stillness. I eventually learned this through guided meditation and biofeedback in the late 1970s—long before triptans and, of course, because of the medical reluctance to seriously comprehend child pain *as pain*. Connected to a different sort of machine, mind to body, I was able to see the tension of my insides by watching my vitals on a monitor, learning to read my body's responses, and willing, learning the power I had, to turn every red light green.

Band-Aid

When I peel open the wrapper of a Band-Aid, the smell reminds me of my big brother's advice once when I fell and cried. "When you hurt yourself, don't cry—get a Band-Aid." I must have been seven or eight at the time, still getting tutored on how to be tough. I felt ashamed of crying. I didn't want to be a wimp.

But what do you bandage when there's no wound?

Painless

When I asked my dad to knock me unconscious, there must have been the germ of hope—perhaps I can attain access to oblivion, ride out the attacks unconscious and away from the overstimulating world. I knew there had to be something more powerful than sleep, or some way I could harness control of that elusive sleep.

I always found it curious that as a kid, when anyone asked "what age would you like to be if you could be any age?" most kids wanted to be older. Now I can see that it makes sense. Kids, even those very well cared for, don't have the greatest freedoms and have little power. I recall many friends dreaming about what it would be like to be 16 and drive, or go to high school and have a boyfriend! So why was I always the only one who wanted to be younger than I already was?

I didn't want to be older. It could be that I already felt I'd missed out on a carefree childhood, watching my family being broken and then fixed by divorce, sitting out and naively imagining, all the while, that painfree children were enjoying every minute of childhood in ways I couldn't.

But honestly, if I could be anything in the world, what would I really rather be? I'd be painless.

Being young means not being able to advocate for your own treatment, so perhaps my friends had the right idea all along. One thing I believed then as strongly as I believe it today is that children should not have to endure unnecessary pain.

Only then, I didn't know that my beliefs could even matter in the great domain of pain.

Faking it

There is much in the discourse dealing with child migraine about the common adult assumption that children will lie about being sick to get out of something they don't want to do.[3] Obviously this is true sometimes, just as it is true of all people (was it really so long ago that you did the same thing?). But the worst part of this obstacle to adult sympathy for child suffering is how ill applied it is in the case of migraine. If we were lying, wouldn't we come up with something more dramatic and convincing than "It's just that my head hurts so bad that I want to die"?

Never mind all the throwing up. They say some bulimics can gag at will—I would guess the reverse is true for many migraineurs: from all the practice with nausea and vomiting some of us are able to prevent the embarrassment of projectile vomiting in public, which is no small feat. Those of us who start getting attacks early get a lot of practice. We can keep the most embarrassing symptoms in control much of the time. I'll spare you the mechanics, but suffice it to say that I can only recall two or three episodes in the past 10 years where I wasn't able to control the vomiting in front of others. But perhaps this is a bad thing—after all, many migraineurs report that vomiting lessens the pain temporarily. Perhaps if child migraineurs trapped in school threw up more, their teachers would have no choice but to help them. Then again, can't we have a little pride left intact?

My brother pronounced me "hyperactive" when I was a kid—very noisy and frenetically moving about. But by my mother's account, when she picked me up from school on migraine days, I lay rigid and unnaturally still across the back seat of the car without even a hint of sound. If you see a young migraineur hitting their head against the wall, you can be sure that they have yet to submit to the terrible truth about this impairment: once an attack begins, it will win. And all the fighting merely escalates the pain and vomiting, as if your body is trying to turn itself inside out in spite of your will, which is punished at the slightest resistance. The migraineur you see lying perfectly still and silent has learned the extraordinary discipline required to *not* writhe in his agony.

Suffering from severe and frequent migraine attacks can define a person in a manner that chases him or her through painfree days as well. My partner, a man who has never complained in spite of countless ER runs in the middle of the night, once made the mistake of trying to console me with the somewhat Hallmarky albeit well-intended statement, "Migraine is a part of who you are." The rage that surged from me at that moment shocked us both as I tried to shout him out of my sight: "It is *no part of me*—it is something that is *done* to me." Not my most eloquent moment, but it rendered an insight about my tappable rage. It comes from decades of blindfolds, tears, wet washcloths, EEGs, MRIs, suspicious doctors, indifferent teachers, homeopathic trial and error, being a pharmaceutical guinea pig, side effects, dry heaves, thunderclaps, lawnmowers, fireworks, sudden strobe effects just when the movie is getting good, and not being sure which was more terrifying—getting up to ask the teacher if I could go to the nurse or puking in front of my classmates.

Changing elementary schools several times to adjust to my health needs meant meeting kids from many different districts, so on my first day in junior high, when the popular but uberkind girl (I know, right?) from a school I'd left a few years before warmly greeted me, I was delighted, until the first thing she said after hello was, "Do you still get those *awful* headaches?" Her pity hurt me.

I am not my migraines.

The scar

As a child I was underweight with a very long torso, so I couldn't fit in a one-piece bathing suit without it sagging all around my waist yet not even reaching up to cover my flat chest, so every time I went swimming, my bikini-exposed belly drew a bit of attention from kids who hadn't learned yet to politely ignore it. I got very tired of people staring at my scar, a jagged line crossing above my belly button all the way around my side to midback, with morbid curiosity, "What *happened* to *you*?" In my early years it may have solicited the story I've already shared with you, which has been retold so often that it is as much a part of me as my name. But eventually I tired of the question and the story, which I replaced with a far more interesting account of how I'd had a sex change (only I didn't understand that such a change would involve stitches nether from my navel, so my lie may have been less convincing than I thought it was at the time). I felt that if someone was going to be so nosy I didn't particularly owe them the truth. The lie was my defense against a slight they didn't mean.

But that damn scar couldn't be talked away.

In third grade I had a teacher who didn't like me, story has it, because my father had mocked her at a parent-teacher conference in which she was demonstrating for a class of adults how to use a multiplication table. My dad's class-clown antics are a common family story. But here's what I remember: one day in health class, somehow this offended teacher had me get up in front of the class to show them my scar. In my memory, though I'm fully aware that I've conflated these events, that was the same day, same moment, that Kenny Fullerton threw up right there in the classroom. As I pulled up my shirt just above the belly to be an obedient lab-specimen freak, Kenny lost his disgusting pink, smelly lunch at my feet. There you have it. No wonder I got a bit of a complex over the scar. It was freakish and made people puke at the mere sight of it.

Of course, the scar is not so freakishly large on a fully grown body with midlife pudges as it must have appeared throughout my skinny, wimpish childhood, when it encircled three-fourths of my waist. But even today, the scar catches doctors off guard. "What happened here?" They never fail to ask and point. And for a moment I see behind their professional mask, an unselfconsciously morbid and scientific curiosity that locks their eyes on my abdomen.

Perhaps I should tattoo an explanation to save myself the trouble:

My birthday suit has been rent
So that now only a bloodless trace remains
Like circumstance's irreversible brand
Holding out as the only wild thing on an otherwise carefully gridded map
Proof that I existed, hurt, and then survived
Because someone loved me and another did his job,
Apparently very well.

Strangely, I cannot be touched there. Even the thought of touching the scar makes me shudder.

In the early 1990s my best friend had a cancerous growth removed from her neck, leaving a tiny scar of which she was nonetheless self-conscious. Finally I understood and shared what my mother had said one day after I came home from the swimming pool fed up with prying eyes, pleading for plastic surgery to remove what my childhood vanity could only see as deformity: "Why would you want to eliminate proof of your survival? Don't you understand? You won."

Our scars bear witness to and offer visible proof of the body's wellspring of self-healing. A strength the lucky runts can claim.

And I'm grateful for that, but it happened almost half a century ago. How much I would have liked for a doctor, nurse, or teacher to understand how much worse migraine has been. But there is no scar for that pain—even though it breaks and breaks against me, it leaves no trace.

Rating pain

You get to be a bit like a trained robot rating your pain. It becomes shorthand in your household. When I get home from work with a slow-starter after a skipped lunch, my partner knows a 1 or 2 means I'll keep functioning for as long as I can, or the attack will progress in spite of the oral then injectable abortive meds to a 3, and if I didn't get them in time, my reluctant plod up the stairs means a 4. An hour later, if I can't keep my antiemetic down but am unwilling to get out of bed to get a suppository dose, that's a 5. Past that I probably won't speak to rate it.

Except once. I was in the infusion room where a neurologist was attempting to abort a four-day attack with intravenous anticonvulsants and hydration. Instead, unthinkably, my pain got even worse. I looked at the nurse pleadingly, 6. Then 7. And in spite of being a grown woman with a headache, right there next to the stoic but kind faces of people fighting cancer getting chemo and an elderly man trying to recover from his stroke, I broke down and cried with my head on my knees.

One doctor claims that "the median pain intensity of a migraine attack is said to be 8" (Daniel 9). But I can't help but think that average is skewed by people who didn't have migraine as kids to broaden the scale. For me 8 would be "uncle." Even worse than that pitiful display in the infusion room. Of course rating your pain on a scale from 1 to 10 is entirely subjective, idiosyncratic, calibrated on the range of your experience with pain. But they do give you a hint, "10 being the worst pain imaginable." And I think I can imagine it, so I don't.

I feel stupefied one day when a pain specialist asks me to rate the pain from my dorsal scapular nerve going "chronic" from a minor car-accident injury (read: dying—thankfully, it no longer conducts any current, or whatever you call that nerve juice of neurons firing). That was not *pain*—just a bothersome neuropathic noise, at times maybe a relentless distraction. He presses for more detail, unsatisfied, so I dig back into my memory: "Sure, it may have brought me to tears out of frustration once or twice." He shows me the kid scale[4] with faces, "See, this one is in tears." We are speaking a different language, doc and I. He's the expert, so I relent, but only halfway, "OK, that's how I felt. But that's still not *pain*."

I was shocked another day to overhear a woman standing just outside of a room where I was waiting for an MRI reporting her pain, in a calm voice, as a 9. I panicked, thinking, "Get that woman a gurney. Stat!" My chest tightened with empathy. She'd spoken the unspeakable number that means only one thing to me: it is the worst days of my childhood—certainly not standing, not speaking; it's what I felt before I lost resolve and rhythmically thwacked my head against the headboard of my bed, all of my body surrendered and motionless except the muscles in my neck (not even the muscles in my eyes would stir), my senses so tender that I felt even the slightest sounds under my kneecaps, then assaulting my stomach. That, to me, is the desperation of 9—giving up because you are helpless.

And as long as I have a say, I will not be there again.

How I found god, hypodermically

The migraines let me be a bit as a teenager, trained by pain to curb my sweet-tooth, quit gymnastics, and avoid a long list of triggers, but one time they never abate is if my body is under some other duress: infection, transitory bugs, erratic sleep. Perhaps the only time I've been grateful for such intrusions is the infection that brought me to god, or triptan, that is. Our introduction was, naturally, painful at first. I was in grad school and I didn't feel well. Some back pain I thought was cramps. But the migraines just wouldn't stop. I wound up at the university health center, crumbled in the urgent care unit; I explained the pain, the nausea, the familiar phonophobia and stabbing light. They took my temperature, raised my shirt to check my organs, and saw the scar. Always the drama of that damn scar. Without discussion I was put into a wheel chair and admitted to the campus hospital. Yes, it was a kidney infection and dangerous for someone with my medical history. I tried to explain in the faint voice my pain would allow, "Fuck the fucking kidneys, help me with my head."

But at least once I was isolated in my little room, a nurse with thin, pursed lips revealed that a prescription for the migraine had already been ordered, and she unsheathed the gleaming solution to all of my woes, sumatriptan (clouds part, heavenly music). It was new that year. Right, I thought, you silly nurse, something designed specifically to "relieve" migraine—like Excedrin Migraine, what a joke (not to mention, when painfree with the luxury of dignity, a bit of an insult).

But not long after the injection I felt a wave of weight spread over my body and through my limbs, as if someone had just covered me with a soft, lead blanket. And the pain briefly worsened, but the fist that was my gut slowly relaxed and opened. The brainstorm was retreating. My arms and legs felt a bit heavy, and I slowly realized that, impossibly, the pain was decreasing—something I had not, in my past 20 years as a migraineur, allowed myself to consider was actually possible as anything but a relaxation fantasy. The attack slowly, simply . . . dissolved.

When people find god, or whatever it is that transforms them, their disposition, their vocabulary for living, birthing a capacity for hope, allowing one to take a breath after years of trickling oxygen, I now knew why they feel "reborn." For me, an unwavering atheist by my early teens, this would be the closest I could come to finding renewed faith by reimagining that pain should not torment a body without purpose or beyond one's control. It was as if I'd been reborn into a new, reasonable head, no longer the runt to be pushed away. Migraine no longer would mean that I must hide from the excruciating light and sound of living. I was no longer trigemony's bitch.

Triptan, this was the god I'd heard so much about,[5] disbelieving those who claimed no doubt. This would safeguard, at least, my dignity. Now a last-ditch hope existed—better yet, once self-injectables became available, I could even control aborting attacks myself. And my 20s were a blast.

ER visits

And yet, managing abortive meds is complicated guesswork. Treat aggressively and you are likely to stop attacks but also take so many triptans that it can't be good for the ticker (or circulation), not to mention the rebound effect. Fail to take a triptan in time, and you risk being left with nothing in your arsenal for the next 24 hours. These are the times that I cave to the basic instinct to escape pain. As an adult, I have options other than lying in bed for three to four days when all else fails. I edge closer to the tipping point toward rescue meds, which on evenings and weekends, are only available in emergency departments (unless you are lucky enough to live in a city with a 24-hour migraine clinic).

"Just to warn you," I phone my partner at work, "I might need a ride to the ER." Legally any doctor who will treat breakthrough pain or intractable migraine with demoral and phenergan shots must confirm that the patient has a driver.

This week was final exams, so I left all the fluorescent lights on for the students (normally I turn off half of them for each class period, subjecting students to the dim atmosphere that a vampire might need). "It was those damn fluorescent beasts," I murmur in a venting moan.

"OK, I need the ER," I decide. It's a difficult surrender, but sometimes I feel an immediate sense of hope that at least temporary relief might be coming. It's enough to give me a last surge of strength to compose myself enough for being seen in public, of course, with the same Tupperware puke bowl I've used since childhood (at some point replaced with bright blue vomit bags you stock up on as an ER regular), not much dignity is left, but at least I keep the moaning and tears in check.

Yet melodrama ensues: "I'm such a freak." Sob. Will concentrates on the road, brilliant by now at avoiding bumps and sharp turns.

"It's a good thing we didn't have kids. I could never do this to another human being."

Patient, quiet, he knows the few sounds I make are painful, and sounds I can't control are even worse. I'm merely feeling sorry for myself, and creating a distraction.

Every time it seems the waiting room is filled with explosive cartoon noise from the television, even if there's no one there to watch it. Sometimes, as if that's not enough, it's accompanied by an assault of country music somehow invading the same space (I live in the Midwest). I tell my partner, "I've read that some people only experience phonophobia or photophobia, but not both." I feel like every sound is magnified and banging inside my skull. The slightest light stabs sharply at the periphery of my vision, prying its way in despite my efforts to keep it out (the sunglasses glued to my face indoors, the squint). "And why, always, does it have to be country? No matter how painful, the Clash would at least be worthy of my effort to grimace through this."

"Phonophobia, photophobia, countriphobia." He recites my symptoms. It takes a saint's tolerance to muster up a sense of humor after so many rescue runs. And patience is in order, because each visit begins with the seemingly innocuous "Have you ever had one of these headaches before?"

Once the nurse has screened against drug-seeking, stroke, and sinus headaches, I'm left in a dark room with my partner, who always brings a book but never reads. The regular rhythm of the clock clangs in my skull, and even the little lamp they've left at a low angle for light seems too much after the sensory onslaught of the waiting room.

It is the same ritual repeated time and again, endured for the chance of relaxing the fist in my gut, a final release from the sense that my body hangs like a puppet from the jerking roughness of a careless god's hand, tense with permanent discomfort.

The doctor tries to make small talk, something I have no room left for in my brain. Always apologetically shining the light right into my eyes, as if to poke where it hurts to find, "Is this it?" Bizarrely, one time the doctor offers: "I like to provide an extra service—would you like for me to say a prayer?" I feel accosted and bullied—in other words, you're a runt, so I can badger you with my god.

I don't care to be polite. *It took everything I had just to tell you my damned story, starting from page one, for probably the twentieth time since I moved to this town* (why don't they use the migraineur profile they suspiciously demanded that my doctor send them, which instructs them to use Nubain?). If a medical doctor thinks his prayer can help me, isn't that a bit like saying it is all in my head? I'm reduced to the role of junkie to pusher, while he doesn't even have to think about treating me as an autonomous, private being with a right to my own godless views. He is treating me like a child, which I now recall, is not such a pleasant thing. I close my eyes to wait for the nurse and remember many harder waits as a child—waiting for a ride home from the noisy chaos of school, waiting for sleep, waiting for what seems to be forever, for relief.

Sleep

Back in the pre-triptan days, and this is still the case for those too young to be treated with prophylactic or abortive meds (and those who have yet to find any effective), the only natural relief for a severe migraine attack was a long and very deep sleep. I still often sleep as long as 16 hours without waking after particularly lengthy and severe attacks, which seems consistent with my memories of some childhood attacks. It feels like hibernating. Getting there is profoundly difficult for child migraineurs (who are more likely to have insomnia, also a possible trigger). Meditation, relaxation therapy, and a slew of homeopathic sleep aids may be tried. But ultimately it all depends upon the body and brain's ability to yield to the netherworld of Morpheus. Once able finally to fall and plunge deeply enough into this world, we may awaken surprised, much later, to a very changed sensory environment. This is the only part of childhood migraine I will ever reflect on fondly—the wonder of waking like Rip Van Winkle alone, to find the enemy has retreated and the world is a quiet, peaceful place. It would seem that much time has passed, by the light. And that light no longer hurts, limbs feel utterly new, breathing is easy. Even the air seems happy. Sometimes accompanied with "lifting feelings"[6] like Alice's, I would carefully rejoin the awake-world incredulous and grateful that the cacophony of pain had vanished, filling me in its place with a floating sense of invincibility I could only imagine others took for granted as "normal" reality. I'd wish this sublime gratitude and joy for all the runts I've known, if only these few moments weren't purchased with hours and hours of helpless pain.

Waiting for sleep

You think of all sorts of things when lying in the dark perfectly conscious but wishing you weren't.

I'm a runt, I'm a runt, kept alive by medicine and love.

I imagine that if I lay on the side opposite the pain, the menace might diffuse itself viscously as if covering a larger surface. That it might even out the pain.

I imagine that I am floating in warm water without effort, feeling sunlight on my face that doesn't hurt my eyes.

I imagine that painlessness is as easy as pressing a button, if I could only find it.

I wonder—if others feel this, how do they endure it? Why isn't everybody screaming?

I imagine that the rest of the world is going about life without me, happily painfree and oblivious to suffering. In fact, I am partly right. Those who suffer generally do so out of sight. It took me decades of countless attacks before I could comprehend I wasn't the only one and found my clan.

But now I know—it can't all be in my head if it's in theirs, too.

Notes

1 Ruth Scott, "'It Hurts Red': A Preliminary Study of Children's Perception of Pain" *Perceptual and Motor Skills* 47 (1978): 787–791.

2 For historical perspective on food dyes and FDA inaction, see Weiss (2012).

3 This presumption underlies every discussion of "pain behavior" I've read. The usual concern is about child *misbehavior* stemming from pain experience, rather than a deeper look at causes – early pain anxiety, bewilderment at what seems like adult indifference, or helplessness in recognizing adult inability to relieve pain, and understandable anger, even rage. My mother wrote in her diary 15 months after my ordeal with untreated kidney infections, sepsis, and encephalitis at the age of three, that they resulted in attempts to manipulate her emotionally: "I think this stems from an experience she had in the hospital. After her operation, while she was very depressed, she became very angry with me . . . blamed me for her pain and told me that because of it, she didn't love me anymore" (diary). When I read this as an adult I was mortified to know how much I'd exacerbated her emotional distress, but I was also impressed that my mother recognized something I have barely seen mentioned in all of my readings about child pain. Sure, kids can be stoic, or sad, but we can also be *angry* about our pain. In spite of my brat attacks, my mother recognized my full emotional agency instead of whitewashing it with a portrait of heroic stoicism or pathetic victimization.

4 Eula Biss writes that the Wong-Baker scale was revised to be more emotionally "neutral" because "several studies have suggested that children using the Wong-Baker scale tend to conflate emotional pain and physical pain" (2007, 34). Numerically, she notes, "Overwhelmingly, patients tend to rate their pain as a five, unless they are in excruciating pain. At best, this renders the scale far less sensitive to gradations in pain. At worst, it renders the scale useless" (35).

5 Hopefully, after the context provided in chapters 2, 3, and 4, this will not sound like a love letter to Glaxo Wellcome.

6 I am borrowing Hustvedt's term here for Alice-in-Wonderland-syndrome perceptions of elongation (2008). Though I recall feeling taller after attacks, it is typically experienced before them.

Postscript: *Child Pain, Migraine, and Invisible Disability* is the result of eight years of reading, six years of interviewing 30 comrades in pain, approximately 300 successfully aborted migraine attacks, and 25 ER visits. No dogs were harmed in the making of this book.

Appendix

Interview questionnaire

Date:
Name:
I prefer to be identified by my real name. _____yes _____no
If no above, what alias would you like to go by?
Email address:
Date of Birth:
Place of Birth:

1 When did your migraines begin (age/year)?

    a   Please describe your strongest memories of early migraine:
    b   How did you respond? How did friends and family respond?
    c   Were you diagnosed and treated medically? If so, please describe.
    d   How did your school respond? Did they help your migraine management during school hours or not? Please be detailed.

2 Do you have aura (visual disturbance, phantom smells) before attacks? If so, please describe.
3 Do you think you have a high tolerance for pain?
4 Have you relied on pain medications (solely or supplemental to triptans)? If so, which?

    a   Have you ever feared addiction?

5 Ever experienced euphoria after attack subsides? If so, please describe.
6 Have you ever developed any superstitions about preventing and relieving migraine?
7 How has migraine affected who you are today? Your personality?
8 Some who are severely impaired have attempted to get disability benefits for migraine. How do you feel about calling migraine a disability?
9 (If adult) how does experiencing migraine as a child differ from adult migraine?
10 What do you wish non-migraineurs understood better?

Works cited

Abu-Arefeh, Ishaq and George Russell. "Prevalence of Headache and Migraine in School-children" *BMJ: British Medical Journal* 309.6957 (Sept. 24, 1994): 765–769.

Acampora, Christa Davis and Ralph R. Acampora. *A Nietzschean Bestiary: Becoming Animal beyond Docile and Brutal*. Lanham, MD: Rowman and Littlefield, 2004.

Adams, Abby. "The Use of Specific Play Techniques in the Treatment of Headaches in Children and Adolescents" in *Headaches in Children*. Eds. Arnold P. Friedman and Ernest Harms. Springfield, IL: Charles C. Thomas, 1967: 131–141.

Adams, Rachel. *Raising Henry: A Memoir of Motherhood, Disability, and Discovery*. New Haven: Yale University Press, 2013.

Albo, Mike. *Hornito: My Lie Life, a Novel*. New York: HarperCollins, 2000.

Alderson, Priscilla. *Children's Consent to Surgery*. Buckingham: Open University Press, 1993.

Alpay, Kadriye, Mustafa Ertas, Elif Kocasoy Orhan, Didem Kanca Ustay, Camille Lieners, and Betül Baykan. "Diet Restriction in Migraine, Based on IgG Against Foods: A Clinical Double-Bind, Randomized, Cross-over Trial" *Cephalalgia* 30 (2010): 829–837.

Alston, Philip. "The Unborn Child and Abortion Under the Draft Convention on the Rights of the Child" *Human Rights Quarterly* 12.1 (Feb. 1990): 156–178.

Anand, K. J. S. and Kenneth D. Craig. "New Perspectives on the Definition of Pain" *Pain* 67 (1996): 3–6.

Anon. "Do Little Bellyachers Grow Up to become Big Bellyachers?" *British Medical Journal* 2.5969 (May 31, 1975): 459–460.

Antilla, Pirjo and Liisa Metsähonkala, Matti Sillanpää. "Long-Term Trends in the Incidence of Headache in Finnish Schoolchildren" *Pediatrics* 117.6 (Jun. 2006): e1197–e2001.

Arnott, Robert. "Surgical Practice in the Prehistoric Aegean" *Medizinhistoriches Journal* 32.3–4 (1997): 249–278.

Aromaa, Minna. "Childhood Headache at School Entry" *Neurology* 50 (1998): 1729–1736.

Aromaa, Minna, Päivi Rautava, Hans Helenius, and Matti L. Sillanpää. "Factors of Early Life as Predictors of Headache in Children at School Entry" *Headache* 38.1 (1998): 23–30.

Ashwal, Stephen, ed. *The Founders of Child Neurology*. San Francisco: Norman Publishing, 1990.

Ask-Upmark, Erik. "Migraine as a Deadly Disease" *British Medical Journal* 2.5202 (Sept. 17, 1960): 823–825.

Aurora, Sheena K., S. H. Kori, P. Barrodale, S. A. McDonald, and D. Haseley. "Gastric Stasis in Migraine: More Than Just a Paroxysmal Abnormality During a Migraine Attack" *Headache* 46 (2006): 57–63.

Avilés, William. Message to the Author. 1 January, 2016. Email.

Bailin, Miriam. *The Sickroom in Victorian Fiction: The Art of Being Ill.* Cambridge: Cambridge University Press, 1994.

Barker, Kristin. "Self-Help Literature and the Making of an Illness Identity: The Case of Fibromyalgia Syndrome (FMS)" *Social Problems* 49.3 (2002): 279–300.

Barlow, Charles F. "Migraine in the Infant and Toddler" *Journal of Child Neurology* 9 (1994): 92–94.

Beah, Ishmael. *A Long Way Gone: Memoirs of a Boy Soldier.* New York: Sarah Crichton Books, 2007.

Beauchard, David. *Epileptic.* New York: Random House, 2005.

Bechdel, Alison. *The Essential Dykes to Watch Out For.* Boston: Houghton Mifflin Harcourt, 2008.

Beil, Laura. "Head Agony: Jumpy Cells May Underlie Migraine's Sensory Storm" *Science News* 181.2 (2012): 26–29.

Bemelmans, Ludwig. *Madeline.* New York: Viking Press, 1939.

Bener, A., S. A. Uduman, E. M. A. Qassimi, G. Khalaily, L. Sztriha, H. Kilpelainen, and E. Obineche. "Genetic and Environmental Factors Associated with Migraine in Schoolchildren" *Headache* 40.2 (Feb. 2000): 152–157.

Bensted, R., D. S. Hargreaves, J. Lombard, U. Kilkelly, and R. M. Viner. "Comparison of Healthcare Priorities in Childhood and Early/Late Adolescence: Analysis of Cross-Sectional Data from Eight Countries in the Council of Europe Child-Friendly Healthcare Survey, 2001" *Child: Care, Health and Development* 41.1 (2014): 160–165.

Benzel, Jessica. Message to the Author. 3 July, 2013. E-mail.

Berde, Charles, Navil F. Sethna, Bruce Masek, Martin Fosburg, and Suzanne Rocklin. "Pediatric Pain Clinics: Recommendations for Their Development" *Paediatrican* 16 (1989): 94–102.

Berger, James. "Falling Towers and Postmodern Wild Children: Oliver Sacks, Don DeLillo, and Turns Against Language" *PMLA* 120.2 (Mar. 2005): 341–361.

Bergman, Thomas. *Moments That Disappear: Children Living with Epilepsy.* Milwaukee: Gareth Stevens Press, 1992.

Bernstein, Robin. *Racial Innocence: Performing American Childhood from Slavery to Civil Rights.* New York: New York University Press, 2011.

Berry, Frederic A. and George A. Gregory. "Do Premature Infants Require Anesthesia?" *Anesthesiology* 67 (1987): 291.

Best, Shaun. "The Social Construction of Pain: An Evaluation" *Disability and Society* 22.2 (Mar. 2007): 161–171.

Bhatt-Mehta, Varsha. "Current Guidelines for the Treatment of Acute Pain in Children" *Drugs* 51.5 (May 1996): 760–776.

Bic, Zuzana, Glen G. Blix, Helen P. Hopp, Frances M. Leslie, and Michael J. Schell. "The Influence of a Low-Fat Diet on Incidence and Severity of Migraine Headaches" *Journal of Women's Health and Gender-Based Medicine* 8.5 (1999): 623–630.

Bille, Bo. "Juvenile Headache: Its Natural History in Children" in *Headaches in Children.* Ed. Arnold P. Friedman. Springfield, Il: Charles C. Thomas, 1967: 10–28.

———. "Migraine in School Children" *Acta Paediatrica* 51.supplement 136 (1962): 1–145.

Birge, Sarah. "No Life Lessons Here: Comics, Autism, and Empathetic Scholarship" *Disability Studies Quarterly* 30.1 (2010). Web.

Bisgaier, M. S. W. and Karin V. Rhodes. "Auditing Access to Speciality Care for Children with Public Insurance" *The New England Journal of Medicine* 364.24 (2011): 2324–2333.

Biss, Eula. *On Immunity: An Inoculation*. Minneapolis: Graywolf, 2014.

———. "The Pain Scale" in *Touchstone Anthology of Contemporary Creative Nonfiction*. Eds. Lex Williford and Michael Martone. New York: Simon and Schuster, 2007: 28–42.

Blaska, Joan K. *Using Children's Literature to Learn about Disabilities and Illness: For Parents and Professionals Working with Young Children*. Troy, NY: Educator's International Press, Inc., 2003.

Blau, J. N. "Fears Aroused in Patients by Migraine" *British Medical Journal* 288.6424 (Apr. 14, 1984): 1126.

Block, James E. *The Crucible of Consent: American Child Rearing and the Forging of Liberal Society*. Cambridge: Harvard University Press, 2012.

Blondin, Betsy Baxter, ed. *Migraine Expressions: A Creative Journey Through Life with Migraine*. Carlsbad, CA: Word Metro Press, 2008.

Bloor, Edward. *Story Time*. Orlando: Harcourt, 2004.

Bluebond-Langner, Myra. *The Private Worlds of Dying Children*. Princeton, NJ: Princeton University Press, 1978.

Bohlmann, Markus. "In Any Event: Moving Rhizomatically in Peter Cameron's Someday This Pain Will be Useful to You" *Children's Literature Association Quarterly* 39.3 (2014): 385–412.

Booth, Martin. *Opium: A History*. New York: St. Martin's Griffin, 1996.

Boswell, John. *The Kindness of Strangers: The Abandonment of Children in Western Europe from Late Antiquity to the Renaissance*. New York: Pantheon, 1988.

Bourke, Joanna. *The Story of Pain: From Prayer to Painkillers*. Oxford: Oxford University Press, 2014.

Bral, Ellen E. "CE Credit: Migraine in Children" *The American Journal of Nursing* 99.11 (Nov. 1999): 35–42.

Breggin, Peter. *Biological Psychiatry vs. Empathy and Human Connection: How Psychiatric Drugs Do More Harm Than Good*. University of Nebraska at Kearney, Ponderosa Room, Student Union. 15 Sept. 2014.

Brennan, Frank, D. B. Carr, and M. Cousins. "Pain Management: A Fundamental Human Right" *Pain Medicine* 105.1 (Jul. 2007): 205–221.

Breslau, Naomi, G. C. Davis, and P. Andreski. "Migraine, Psychiatric Disorders, and Suicide Attempts: An Epidemiologic Study of Young Adults" *Psychiatry Research* 37 (1991): 11–23.

Brewster, Arlene B. "Chronically Ill Hospitalized Children's Concept of Their Illness" *Pediatrics* 69.3 (Mar. 1982): 355–362.

Bridgeman, Jo. "The Child's Body" in *Real Bodies: A Sociological Introduction*. Eds. Mary Evans and Ellie Lee. Hampshire: Palgrave, 2002: 96–114.

Brummer, Anna. Personal Interview. 5 May, 2011.

Bulkagov, Mikhail. *The Master and Margarita*. Trans. Diana Burgin and Katherine O'Connor. New York: Random House, 1996.

Burton, Tess. "Painful Memories: Chronic Pain as a Form of Re-Membering" *Memory Studies* 4.23 (2011): 23–32.

Cameron, Hector Charles. *The Nervous Child*. 3rd ed. London: Oxford University Press, 1922.

Camus, Albert. *Exile and the Kingdom*. 1957. Trans. Carol Cosman. New York: Random House, 2007.

————. *The Plague*. 1947. Trans. Stuart Gilbert. New York: Modern Library, 1948.

Canguilhem, Georges. *The Normal and the Pathological*. 1978. Trans. Carolyn R. Fawcett. New York: Zone Books, 1991.

Cantor, Carla and Brian Fallon. *Phantom Illness: Shattering the Myth of Hypochondria*. Boston: Houghton Mifflin, 1996.

Carroll, Lewis. *Alice's Adventures Under Ground*. 1864. London: Pavilion Books, 1985.

————. *The Annotated Alice*. Ed. Martin Gardner. New York: Meridian, 1960.

Cassel, Eric J. *The Nature of Suffering: And the Goals of Medicine*. New York: Oxford University Press, 1991.

Cate, Curtis. *Friedrich Nietzsche*. New York: The Overlook Press, 2002.

Chakravarty, A. and A. Sen. "Migraine, Neuropathic Pain and Nociceptive Pain: Toward a Unifying Concept" *Medical Hypotheses* 74 (2010): 225–231.

Chambers, Christine. *It Doesn't Have to Hurt*. Tedx Mount Allison University. 16 Jun. 2014. Web. 8 Mar. 2016.

Chaney, Michael A. "The Animal Witness of the Rwandan Genocide" in *Graphic Subjects: Critical Essays on Autobiography and Graphic Novels*. Ed. Michael E. Chaney. Madison: University of Wisconsin Press, 2011: 93–100.

Chang, Ha-Joon. *23 Things They Don't Tell You about Capitalism*. New York: Bloomsbury Press, 2010.

Chen, Mel Y. *Animacies: Biopolitics, Racial Mattering, and Queer Affect*. Durham: Duke University Press, 2012.

————. "Brain Fog: The Race for Cripistemology" *Journal of Literary and Cultural Disability Studies* 8.2 (2014): 171–184.

Chilman-Blair, Kim and Shawn deLoache. *Medikidz Explain Chronic Pain: What's Up with Moira's Grandad?* London: Medikidz Limited, 2012.

Churchland, Patricia S. *Touching a Nerve: The Self as Brain*. New York: W. W. Norton, 2013.

Cioffi, Frank L. "Graphic Fictions on Graphic Subjects: Teaching the Illustrated Medical Narrative" in *Teaching the Graphic Novel*. Ed. Stephen Ely Tabachnick. New York: MLA of America, 2009: 179–187.

Clark, Anna. "Krazy Komic" *Guernica: A Magazine of Art and Politics*. Oct. 23, 2014. Downloaded Oct. 1, 2013. www.guernicamag.com/features/krazy-komic/

Clark, Cindy Dell. *In Sickness and Play: Children Coping with Chronic Illness*. New Brunswick: Rutgers University Press, 2003.

Coakley, Sarah and Kay Kaufman Shelemay, eds. *Pain and Its Transformations: The Interface of Biology*. Cambridge: Harvard University Press, 2007.

Coats, Karen. *Looking Glasses and Neverlands: Lacan, Desire, and Subjectivity in Children's Literature*. Iowa City: University of Iowa Press, 2004.

Cohen, Esther. "The Expression of Pain in the Middle Ages: Deliverance, Acceptance and Infamy" in *Bodily Extremities: Preoccupations with the Human Body in Early European Culture*. Eds. Florike Egmond and Robert Zwijnenberg. Burlington, VT: Ashgate 2003: 195–219.

Cohen, Morton N. *Lewis Carroll: A Biography*. New York: Alfred A. Knopf, 1995.

Coolidge, Susan. *What Katy Did*. 1872. New York: Puffin Penguin, 1995.

Coren, Stanley. *The Left-Hander Syndrome: The Causes and Consequences of Left-Handedness*. New York: The Free Press, 1992.

Cornock, Marc and Heather Montgomery. "Children's Rights In and Out of the Womb" *International Journal of Children's Rights* 19 (2011): 3–19.

Courtwright, David, Herman Joseph, and Don Des Jarlais. *Addicts Who Survived: An Oral History of Narcotic Use in America: 1923–1965*. Knoxville: University of Tennessee Press, 1989.

Couser, G. Thomas. *Vulnerable Subjects: Ethics and Life Writing*. Ithaca: Cornell University Press, 2004.

Cousins, Michael J. "Relief of Acute Pain: A Basic Human Right?" *Medical Journal of Australia* 172 (2000): 3–4.

Cousins, Michael J., F. Brennan F, and D. B. Carr DB. "Pain Relief: A Universal Human Right" *Pain* 112 (2004): 1–4.

Cowie, Dorothy, Tamar R. Makin, and Andrew J. Bremmer. "Children's Responses to the Rubber-Hand Illusion Reveal Dissociable Pathways in Body Representation" *Psychological Science* 24.5 (2013): 762–769.

Crain, Patricia. "Regarding the Pain of Children" *American Literary History* 25.2 (2013): 418–429.

Crockett, Annecy. Personal Interview. 2 January, 2013.

———. Personal Interview. 1 May, 2014.

———. Unpublished Diary. December, 2013.

Crockett, Carrie. Personal Interview. 1 May, 2014.

———. 11 November 2014. Email.

Crow, Carolyn S. "Children's Pain Perspectives Inventory (CCPI): Development Assessment" *Pain* 72 (1997): 33–40.

Dahler, Michel. "Pain Relief is a Human Right" *Asian Pacific Journal of Cancer Prevention* 11 (2010): 97–101.

Damasio, Antonio. "How the Brain Creates the Mind" *Scientific American*. 12.1. (Dec. 1999): 112–117.

Daniel, Britt Talley. *Migraine*. Bloomington: Author House, 2010.

Darling-Hammond, Linda. *The Flat World and Education: How America's Commitment to Equity Will Determine Our Future*. New York: Teacher's College Press, 2010.

Davis, Lennard. "Bodies of Difference: Politics, Disability, and Representation" in *Disability Studies: Enabling the Humanities*. Eds. Sharon L. Snyder, Brenda Jo Brueggemann, and Rosemarie Garland-Thomson. New York: Modern Language Association, 2002: 100–106.

———, ed. *The Disability Studies Reader*. 4th ed. New York: Routledge, 2013.

———. "Life, Death, and Biocultural Literacy" *The Chronicle Review*. 6 Jan. 2006. Web. 10 May 2015.

Davis, N. Ann. "Invisibility Disability" *Ethics* 116.1 (2005): 153–213.

Davis, Terrell with Adam Schefter. *TD: Dreams in Motion*. New York: HarperCollins, 1998.

Dawkins, Richard. *The Selfish Gene*. Oxford: Oxford University Press, 1989.

de Almeida, R. F. and P. A. Kowacs. "Anne Frank's Headache" *Cephalalgia* 27 (2007): 1215–1218.

DeJong, Russell N. "The Causes and Treatments of Headaches" *The American Journal of Nursing* 55.1 (Jan. 1955): 54–58.

Dengler, Regina and Heather Roberts. "Adolescents Use of Prescribed Drugs and Over-the-Counter Preparations" *Journal of Popular Medicine* 18.4 (1996): 437–442.

Desmon, Stephanie. "Blood Levels of Fat Cell Hormone May Predict Severity of Migraines" *Johns Hopkins Medicine*. 18 Mar. 2013. Web. 11 Dec. 2015.

Didion, Joan. "In Bed" 1968. in *The White Album*. New York: Simon and Schuster, 1979: 168–172.

Diller, Lawrence. *The Last Normal Child: Essays on the Intersection of Kids, Culture, and Psychiatric Drugs*. Westport, CT: Praeger, 2006.

DiMario, Francis J., Jr. "Childhood Headaches: A School Nurse Perspective" *Clinical Pediatrics* 31.5 (May 1992): 279–282.

Dodick, David and Stephen Silberstein. "Central Sensitization Theory of Migraine: Clinical Implications" *Headache* 46.4 (2006): S182–S191.

Donadey, Anne. "Representing Gender and Sexual Trauma: Moufida Tlatli's *Silences of the Palace*" *South Central Review* 28.1 (2011): 36–51.

Dooley, Joseph, Kevin Gordon, and Peter Carnfield. "The Rushes: A Migraine Variant with Hallucinations of Time" *Clinical Pediatrics* 29 (1990): 536–538.

Duane, Anna Mae. *Suffering Childhood in Early America: Violence, Race, and the Making of the Child Victim*. Athens: University of Georgia Press, 2010.

Dumit, Joseph. *Picturing Personhood: Brain Scans and Biomedical Identity*. Princeton: Princeton University Press, 2004.

Dupierris, Martial. "Reduction of a Femoral Dislocation, of Six Months Standing, by Manipulation" *The North American Medicochirgurical Review* 1 (1857): 290–294.

Eadie, Mervyn J. *Headache: Through the Centuries*. New York: Oxford University Press, 2012.

Eberly, Susan Schoon. "Fairies and the Folklore of Disability: Changelings, Hybrids, and the Solitary Fairy" in *The Good People: New Fairylore Essays*. Ed. Peter Narváez. Lexington: University of Kentucky Press, 1991: 227–250.

Eccleston, Christopher and Peter Malleson. "Managing Chronic Pain in Children and Adolescents: We Need to Address the Embarrassing Lack of Data for This Common Problem" *British Medical Journal* 326.7404 (Jun. 28, 2003): 1408–1409.

Edwards, Laurie. *In the Kingdom of the Sick: A Social History of Chronic Illness in America*. New York: Walker and Company, 2013.

Ehrenreich, Barbara and Deidre English. *For Her Own Good: 150 Years of the Experts' Advice to Women*. New York: Anchor-Doubleday, 1978.

Ekman, Paul. *Why Kids Lie: How Parents Can Encourage Truthfulness*. New York: Penguin, 1989.

Elithorn, Alick. "Migraine" *The British Medical Journal* 4.5680 (Nov. 15, 1969): 411–413.

Ellis, Deborah. *No Ordinary Day*. Toronto: Groundwood Books, 2011.

Emminghaus, Wolf B., Paul R. Kimmel, and Edward C. Stewart. "Primal Violence: Illuminating Culture's Dark Side" in *The Handbook of Interethnic Coexistence*. Ed. Eugene Weiner. New York: Continuum, 1998: 126–149.

Endebrock, Tyler. "Cardale Jones Hospitalized with Severe Head Pain" *The Sports Quotient*. 2 Sept. 2015. Web. 2 Sept. 2015.

Enders, Giulia. *Gut: The Inside Story of Our Body's Most Underrated Organ*. Vancouver: Greystone, 2015.

Espir, Michael, L. E. Espir, I. L. Hodge, and P. H. Matthews. "Footballer's Migraine" *The British Medical Journal* 3.5822 (Aug. 5, 1972): 352.

Feldman, Marc D. *Playing Sick? Untangling the Web of Munchausen Syndrome, Munchausen by Proxy, Malingering, and Factious Disorder*. New York: Routledge, 2004.

Fensch, Thomas. *Alice in Acidland*. The Woodlands, TX: New Century Books, 1970.

———. "Lewis Carroll – the First Acidhead" 1968. in *Aspects of Alice: Lewis Carroll's Dreamchild as Seen Through the Critics' Looking-Glasses*. Ed. Robert Phillips. New York: Vanguard Press, 1971.

Fields, R. Douglas. *The Other Brain: From Dementia to Schizophrenia, How New Discoveries about the Brain Are Revolutionizing Medicine and Science*. New York: Simon and Schuster, 2009.

Fiering, Greg. *I Don't Love You! The Best of Migraine Boy*. San Jose: SLG Publishing, 2004.

Firestone, Shulamith. *The Dialectic of Sex: The Case for Feminist Revolution.* New York: William Morrow and Company, 1970.

Fishman, Scott and Lisa Berger. *The War on Pain.* New York: HarperCollins, 2001.

Flanagan, Bob. *The Pain Journal.* Los Angeles: Smart Art Press, 2000.

Fleming, Thomas. *Duel: Alexander Hamilton, Aaron Burr, And The Future Of America.* New York: Basic Books, 1999.

Flor, Herta and Niels Birbaumer. "Acquisition of Chronic Pain: Psychophysiological Mechanisms" *APS Journal* 3.2 (1994): 119–127.

Foreman, Judy. *A Nation in Pain: Healing Our Nation's Biggest Health Problem.* Oxford: Oxford University Press, 2014.

Forlag, Vilhelm Trydes. "Primitive Trephining" *The British Medical Journal* 2.2900 (Jul. 29, 1916): 150–151.

Fortuine, Robert. "Lancets of Stone: Traditional Methods of Surgery among the Alaska Natives" *Artic Anthropology* 22.1 (1985): 23–45.

Fox, Marie and Michael Thomson. "Short Changed? The Law and Ethics of Male Circumcision" *The International Journal of Children's Rights* 13 (2005): 161–181.

Frank, Anne. *The Diary of Anne Frank: The Revised Critical Edition.* Eds. David Barnouw and Gerrold Van Der Stroom. New York: Doubleday, 1989.

Frank, Arthur W. *At the Will of the Body: Reflections on Illness.* New York: Houghton Mifflin, 2002.

———. *The Wounded Storyteller: Body, Illness, and Ethics.* Chicago: University of Chicago Press, 1995.

Frank, Lone. *Midfield: How Brain Science Is Changing Our World.* Oxford: One World, 2009.

Frazer, James George. *The New Golden Bough: A New Abridgement of the Classic Work.* New York: Criterion, 1959.

Frederick, Leon. Message to the Author. 9 August, 2014. E-mail.

———. Personal Interview. 18 October, 2013.

Freedman, Ariela. "Sorting Through My Grief and Putting It into Boxes: Comics and Pain" in *Knowledge and Pain.* Eds. Esther Cohen, Leona Tucker, Manuela Consonni, and Otniel E. Dror. Amsterdam: Rodopi, 2012: 381–399.

French, Renée. *H Day.* Brooklyn: Picturebox, 2010.

———. Strand Bookstore. "H Day" updated 14 Dec. 2010. YouTube. Web. 18 Aug. 2013.

Friedman, Arnold P. "The Headache in History, Literature, and Legend" *Bulletin of the New York Academy of Medicine* 48.4 (1972): 661–681.

Fudge, Erica. *Animal.* London: Reaktion, 2002.

Fulda, Jennette. *Chocolate and Vicodin: My Quest for Relief from the Headache That Wouldn't Go Away.* New York: Gallery Books, 2011.

Gafney, Anne and Elizabeth A. Dunne. "Children's Understanding of the Causality of Pain" *Pain* 29 (1987): 91–94.

Galdós, Benito Pérez. *Forunata and Jacinta: Two Stories of Married Women.* 1886–1887. Trans. Agnes Moncy Gullón. New York: Penguin, 1988.

Gall, Robert. Personal Interview. 26 April, 2015.

Garland-Thomson, Rosemarie. *Staring: How We Look.* Oxford: Oxford University Press, 2009.

Garma, Angel. "Jaquea, Seudo-Oligofrenia y Delirio en un Personaje de Pérez Galdós" *Ficción.* 14 (1958): 84–102.

Gershon, Michael D. *The Second Brain: The Scientific Basis of Gut Instinct and a Groundbreaking New Understanding of Nervous Disorders of the Stomach and Intestine.* New York: HarperCollins, 1998.

Gilbert, Carlean M. "Coping with Pediatric Migraine: Differences between Copers and Non-Copers" *Child and Adolescent Social Work Journal* 12.4 (1995): 275–287.

Goedert, Dee. Personal Interview. 17 April, 2011.

Goffman, Erving. *Stigma: Notes on the Management of Spoiled Identity*. Englewood Cliffs: Prentice Hall, 1963.

Golden, Gerald S. "The Alice in Wonderland Syndrome in Juvenile Migraine" *Pediatrics* 63 (1979): 517–519.

Good, Peter. A., Rod S. Taylor, and M. J. Mortimer. "The Use of Tinted Glasses in Childhood Migraine" *Headache* 31 (1991): 533–536.

Goodacre, Selwyn H. "The Illness of Lewis Carroll" *The Practitioner* 209 (1972): 230–239.

Gordon, Lyndall. *Lives Like Loaded Guns: Emily Dickinson and Her Family's Feuds*. New York: Penguin, 2010.

Grant, Vicki. *Triggered*. Victoria: Orca, 2013.

Gregory, Julie. *Sickened: The Memoir of a Munchausen by Proxy Childhood*. New York: Bantam, 2003.

Green, Katie. *Lighter Than My Shadow*. London: Jonathan Cape, 2013.

Green, Sara E. "Staying True to Their Stories: Interviews with Parents of Children with Disabilities" in *Disability and Qualitative Inquiry: Methods for Rethinking an Ableist World*. Eds. Ronald Berger and Laura S. Lorenz. Burlington: Ashgate, 2–15, 2015: 57–73.

Greenberg, Joel. "The Lore of Cocaine" *Science News* 114.11 (Sept. 9, 1978): 187–188, 191.

Griffiths, Niall. *Runt*. London: Routledge, 2007.

Grinspoon, Lester and James B. Bakalar. *Marihuana, the Forbidden Medicine*. New Haven: Yale University Press, 1993.

Grof, Stanislav. "Stanislav Grof Interviews Dr. Albert Hoffmann" 1984. *Maps* 11.2 (2011): 22–35.

Grøholt, Else-Karin, Hein Stigum, Rannveig Nordhagen, and Lennart Köhler. "Recurrent Pain in Children, Socio-Economic Factors and Accumulation in Families" *European Journal of Epidemiology* 18 (2003): 965–975.

Gross, Charles G. "A Hole in the Head" *History of Neuroscience* 5 (1999): 263–269.

Gross, Jane. "Camp Fixtures" *New York Times*. Jul. 16, 2006. Web. Downloaded May 19, 2014.

Grossinger, Richard. *Migraine Auras: When the Visual World Fails*. Berkeley: North Atlantic Books, 2006.

Grosz, Elizabeth. *Volatile Bodies: Toward a Corporeal Feminism*. Bloomington: Indiana University Press, 1994.

Gwyther, Liz, Frank Brennan, and Richard Harding. "Advancing Palliative Care as a Human Right" *Journal of Pain and Symptom Management* 38.5 (2009): 767–774.

Haan, Joost. "Migraine and Metaphor" *Frontiers of Neurology and Neuroscience* 31 (2013): 126–136.

———. Personal Interview. 8 July, 2015.

Haas, David C. and Robert D. Sovner. "Migraine Attacks Triggered by Mild Head Trauma, and Their Relation to Certain Post-Traumatic Disorders of Childhood" *Journal of Neurology and Neurosurgery* 32 (1969): 548–554.

Hacker, Marilyn. "Migraine Sonnets" in *The Paris Review Book of Heartbreak, Madness, Sex, Love, Betrayal, Outsiders, Intoxication, War, Whimsy, Horrors, God, Death, Dinner, Baseball, Travels, the Art of Writing, and Everything Else in the World Since 1953*. New York: Picador, 2003: 188–189.

Hagger, Lynne and Simon Woods. "Children and Research: A Risk of Double Jeopardy?" *The International Journal of Children's Rights* 13 (2005): 51–72.

Hall, Carrie. Telephone Interview. 17 December, 2014.

Hampton, Tracy. "Experts Weigh in on Promotion, Prescription of Off-Label Drugs" *JAMA* 297.7 (2007): 683–684.

Hansen, Bert. "Medical History for the Masses: How American Comic Books Celebrated Heroes of Medicine in the 1940s" *Bulletin of the History of Medicine* 78.1 (2004): 148–191.

Haraway, Donna. *The Companion Species Manifesto: Dogs, People, and Significant Otherness*. Chicago: Prickly Paradigm Press, 2003.

Harris, Gemma Elwin, ed. *Big Questions from Little People and Simple Answers from Great Minds*. New York: HarperCollins, 2012.

Harrison, Helen. "Letters to the Editor" *Birth* 13 (1986): 124–125.

Hartley, David. *Observations on Man, His Frame, His Duty, and His Expectations*. 1749. Facsimile reproduction. Gainesville, FL: Scholar's Facsimiles and Reprints, 1966.

Harvey, Cedric C. "Abdominal Migraine in Children" *The British Medical Journal* 1.4980 (Jun. 16, 1956): 1429–1430.

Harwood, Rowan H., Avan Aihie Sayer, and Miriam Hirschfeld. "Current and Future Worldwide Prevalence of Dependency, Its Relationship to Total Population, and Dependency Ratios" *Bulletin of World Health Organization* 82 (2004): 251–258.

Hawkins, Anne Hunsaker. "Writing about Illness: Therapy? or Testimony?" in *Unfitting Stories: Narrative Approaches to Disease, Disability, and Trauma*. Eds. Valerie Raoul, Connie Canam, and Angela D Henderson. Waterloo, Ontario: Wilfrid Laurier University Press, 2007: 113–127.

Hering-Hanit, R. and N. Gadoth. "Caffeine-induced Headache in Children and Adolescents" *Cephalalgia* 23.5 (2003): 332–335.

Hermes, Patricia. *What if They Knew?* New York: Harcourt, Brace, Jovanovich, 1980.

Hernandez-Latorre, M. A. and M. Roig. "Natural History of Migraine in Childhood" *Cephalalgia* 20 (2000): 573–579.

Hershey, Andrew D. "Refractory Headaches in Children and Adolescents" in *Refractory Migraine: Mechanisms and Management*. Eds. Elliott A. Schulman, Morris Levin, Alvin E. Lake III, and Elizabeth Loder. Oxford: Oxford University Press, 2010: 257–265.

Higgins, Kathleen Marie. *Comic Relief: Nietzsche's Gay Science*. New York: Oxford University Press, 2000.

Hill, William. "On Some Causes of Backwardness and Stupidity in Children" *The British Medical Journal* 2.1500 (Sept. 28, 1889): 711–712.

Hines, Edgar A., Jr. "Migraine" *The American Journal of Nursing* 38.9 (1938): 988–992.

Hofmann, Albert. *LSD, My Problem Child: Reflections on Sacred Drugs, Mysticism, and Science*. 1979. Trans. Jonathan Ott. Los Angeles: J. P. Tarcher, 1983.

Hoffman, Beatrix. *Health Care for Some: Rights and Rationing in the United States since 1930*. Chicago: University of Chicago Press, 2012.

Holmes, Anthony. Personal Interview. 15 October, 2014.

Holmes, Jamie. Personal Interview. 26 July, 2015.

Holmes, Lily. Personal Interview. 26 July, 2015.

Honeyman, Mary. Diary. 23 September, 1971.

Hood, Caleb. Personal Interview. 9 March, 2016.

Hrdy, Sarah Blaffer. *Mothers and Others: The Evolutionary Origins of Mutual Understanding*. Cambridge: Harvard University Press, 2009.

Humphrey, Jill C. "Researching Disability Politics, or, Some Problems with the Social Model in Practice" *Disability and Society* 15.1 (2000): 63–85.

Humphrey, Patrick P. A. "The Discovery and Development of Triptans, a Major Therapeutic Breakthrough" *Headache* 48 (2008): 685–687.

Hurley, Alfred and Elaine G. Whelan. "Cognitive Development and Children's Perception of Pain" *Pediatric Nursing* 14.1 (1988): 21–24.

Hustvedt, Siri. "Lifting, Lights, and Little People" *The New York Times*. 17 Feb. 2008. Web. 8 Jun. 2011.

———. "My Strange Head: Notes on Migraine" in *Living, Thinking, Looking: Essays*. New York: Picador, 2012: 24–36.

Iacoboni, Marco. *Mirroring People: The Science of Empathy and How We Connect with Others*. New York: Picador, 2009.

Illich, Ivan. *Limits to Medicine: Medical Nemesis: The Expropriation of Health*. London: Marion Boyars, 1976.

Isenker, Jan. Personal Interview. 23 December, 2014.

Jackson, Jean E. "After a While No One Believes You: Real and Unreal Pain" in *Pain as Human Experience: An Anthropological Perspective*. Eds. Mary-Jo Delveccio, Paul E. Brodwin, Byron J. Good, Arthur Kleinman. Berkeley: University of California Press, 1992: 138–168.

———. "Stigma, Liminality, and Chronic Pain: Mind-Body Borderlands" *American Ethnologist* 32.3 (Aug. 2005): 332–353.

Janeti, Joseph and John C. Liebeskind. "A Call for National Initiatives on Pain" *Pain* 59 (1994): 5–6.

Jaques, Zoe. *Children's Literature and the Posthuman: Animal, Environment, Cyborg*. New York: Routledge, 2015.

Jillian, Susan. "That Beautiful Somewhere – Accurate Depiction of Migraine – as Well as a Great Story" Dec. 2, 2007. http://drupal.ziggurt.com. Web. 22 May 2015.

Johnson, Chloé. Personal Interview. 8 November, 2013.

Johnson, Harriet McBryde. *Accidents of Nature*. New York: Henry Holt & Co., 2006.

———. *Too Late to Die Young: Nearly True Tales from a Life*. New York: Henry Holt & Co., 2005.

———. "Unspeakable Conversations" *New York Times Magazine*. 16 Feb. 2003. www.nytimes.com/2003/02/16/magazine/unspeakable-conversations.html

Jones, Gerard. *Killing Monsters: Why Children Need Fantasy, Super Heroes, and Make-Believe Violence*. New York: Basic Books, 2002.

Jones, Maggie. *Your Child: Headaches and Migraine*. Shatsbury, Dorset: Element, 1999.

Joy, Melanie. *Why We Love Dogs, Eat Pigs, and Wear Cows: An Introduction to Carnism, the Belief System That Enables Us to Eat Some Animals and Not Others*. San Francisco: Conari Press, 2010.

Kabbouche, Marielle A., Anna-Liisa Bentti Vockell, Susan L. LeCates, Scott W. Powers, and Andrew D. Hershey. "Tolerability and Effectiveness of Prochlorperazine for Intractable Migraine in Children" *Pediatrics* 107 (2001): e62.

Kafer, Alison. *Feminist, Queer, Crip*. Bloomington: Indiana University Press, 2013.

Kamen, Paula. *All in My Head, an Epic Quest to Cure and Unrelenting, Totally Unreasonable, and Only Slightly Enlightening Headache*. Cambridge, MA: Da Capo Press, 2005.

Kandall, Stephen R. *SubStance and Shadow: Women and Addiction in the United States*. Cambridge: Harvard University Press, 1996.

Kaplaw, Lawrence. "Distractions Dir. Daniel Attias" *House M.D.* 2.12 (Feb. 14, 2006).

Karasik, Judy and Paul Karasik. *The Ride Together: A Brother and Sister's Memoir of Autism in the Family*. New York: Washington Square Press, 2003.

Kästner, Erich. *Annaluise and Anton.* Trans. Eric Sutton. New York: Dodd, Mead, and Co., 1933.

Kaufman, Eleanor. "Toward a Feminist Philosophy of the Mind" in *Deleuze and Feminist Theory.* Eds. Ian Buchanan and Clair Colebrook. Edinburgh: Edinburgh University Press, 2000: 128–143.

Keen, Suzanne. "Fast Tracks to Narrative Empathy: Anthropomorphism and Dehumanization in Graphic Narratives" *SubStance* 40.1 (2011): 135–155.

Keith, Lois. *Take Up Thy Bed and Walk: Death, Disability, and Cure in Classic Fiction for Girls.* New York: Routledge, 2001.

Kempner, Joanna. *Not Tonight: Migraine and the Politics of Gender and Health.* Chicago: University of Chicago Press, 2014.

Kidd, Kenneth B. *Freud in Oz: At the Intersections of Psychoanalysis and Children's Literature.* Minneapolis: University of Minnesota Press, 2011.

Kilkelly, Ursula and Mark Donnelly. "Participation in Healthcare: The Views and Experiences of Children and Young People" *International Journal of Children's Rights* 19 (2011): 107–125.

Kilkelly, Ursula and Eileen Savage. "Legal and Ethical Dimensions of Communicating with Children and Their Families" in *Communication Skills for Children's Nurses.* Eds. Veronica Lambert, Tony Long, and Deirdre Kelleher. New York: Open University Press, 2012: 137–151.

Kilty, T., N. Charney, and A. Leviton. "Headaches, Performance in High School, and Handedness" *Perceptual and Motor Skills* 65 (1987): 159–163.

Klossowski, Pierre. *Nietzsche and the Vicious Circle.* 1969. Trans. Daniel W. Smith. Chicago: University of Chicago Press, 1997.

Koehler, P. J. and H. Isler. "The Early Use of Ergotamine in Migraine. Edward Woakes' Report of 1868, Its Theoretical and Practical Background and Its International Reception" *Cephalalgia* 22 (2002): 686–691.

Koerth-Baker, Maggie. "The Not-So-Hidden Cause Behind the A.D.H.D. Epidemic" *The New York Times.* Oct. 15, 2013. Web. Downloaded May 19, 2014.

Kohn, Alfie. *Feel-Bad Education and Other Contrarian Essays on Children and Schooling.* Boston: Beacon Press, 2011.

Korczak, Janusz. *Ghetto Diary.* Intro. by Betty Jean Lifton. New Haven: Yale University Press, 1978.

Kramer, Stanley (dir.) and Herman Wouk. *The Caine Mutiny.* 1954. Culver City, Calif.: Sony Pictures Home Entertainment, 2007.

Krane, Elliot J. with Deborah Mitchell. *Relieve Your Child's Chronic Pain.* New York: Simon and Schuster, 2005.

Kuhn, Reinhard. *Corruption in Paradise: The Child in Western Literature.* Hanover: Brown University Press, 1982.

Kuhse, Helga and Peter Singer. *Should the Baby Live? The Problem of Handicapped Infants.* Oxford: Oxford University Press, 1985.

Kuppers, Petra. "Bodies, Hysteria, Pain" in *Bodies in Commotion: Disability and Performance.* Eds. Carrie Sandahl and Philip Auslander. Ann Arbor: University of Michigan Press, 2005: 147–162.

———. *The Scar of Visibility: Medical Performances and Contemporary Art.* Minneapolis: University of Minnesota Press, 2007.

Kuttner, Leora. *A Child in Pain: What Health Professionals Can Do to Help.* Carmarthen, Wales: Crown House Publishing, 2010.

Lack, Dorothea Z. "Women and Pain: Another Feminist Issue" *Women and Therapy* 1.1 (Spring 1982): 55–64.

Ladd, Paddy. *Understanding Deaf Culture: In Search of Deafhood*. Bristol: Multilingual Matters, 2003.

Langeveld, J. H., H. M. Koot, M. C. Loonen, A. A. Hazebroek-Kampschreur, and J. Passchier. "A Quality of Life Instrument for Adolescents with Chronic Headache" *Cephalalgia* 16 (1996): 183–196.

Larner, A. J. "Lewis Carroll's Humpty Dumpty: And Early Report of Prosopagnosia?" *Journal of Neurology, Neurosurgery, and Psychiatry* 75 (2004): 1063.

Larsen, Kevin S. "The Medical Background of *Fortunata y Jacinta*: The Case of Maxi's Migraines" *Ometeca* 3–4 (1996): 410–425.

Lawson, Jill. "Letters to the Editor" *Birth* 13 (1986): 124–125.

Lears, Laurie. *Becky the Brave: A Story about Epilepsy*. Illus. by Gail Piazza. Morton Grove, IL: Albert Whitman and Co., 2002.

Lederer, Susan E. *Subjected to Science: Human Experimentation in America before the Second World War*. Baltimore: Johns Hopkins University Press, 1995.

Leiter, Valerie. *Their Time Has Come: Youth with Disabilities on the Cusp of Adulthood*. New Brunswick: Rutgers University Press, 2012.

Lerner, D. J., B. C. Amick III, S. Malspeis, W. H. Rogers, N. C. Santanello, W. C. Gerth, and R. B. Lipton. "The Migraine Work and Productivity Loss Questionnaire: Concepts and Design" *Quality of Life Research* 8.8 (Dec. 1999): 688–710.

Levy, Andrew. *A Brain Wider Than the Sky: A Migraine Diary*. New York: Simon and Schuster, 2009.

Lewis, D. W., M. T. Middlebrook, L. Mehallick, T. M. Rauch, C. Deline, and E. F. Thomas. "Pediatric Headaches: What Do the Children Want?" *Headache* 36.4 (1996): 224–230.

Lippmann, Caro W. "Certain Hallucinations Peculiar to Migraine" *Journal of Nervous and Mental Disease* 116 (1952): 346–351.

Lipscombe, S. L. and T. Prior. "Is There Any Relationship between Handedness and Unilateral Headache in Migraine?" *Cephalalgia* 22 (2002): 146–148.

Lipski, Elizabeth. *Digestive Wellness*. 4th ed. New York: McGraw Hill, 2012.

Lipton, Richard B. "Diagnosis and Epidemiology of Pediatric Migraine" *Current Opinion in Neurology* 10 (1997): 231–236.

Lisowski, F. P. "Prehistoric and Early Historic Trepanation" in *Diseases in Antiquity: A Survey of the Diseases, Injuries, and Surgery of Early Populations*. Eds. Don Brothwell and A. T. Sandison. Springfield, IL: Charles C. Thomas, 1967: 651–672.

Liveing, Edward. *On Megrim, Sick-Headache, and Some Allied Disorders: A Contribution to the Pathology of Nerve-Storms*. London: J & A Churchill, 1873.

Lloyd-Thomas, A. R. "Pain Management in Paediatric Patients" *British Journal of Anesthesia* 64 (1990): 85–104.

Loder, Elizabeth and David Biondi. "A Disease Modification in Migraine: A Concept That Has Come of Age?" *Headache* 43 (2003): 135–143.

———. "Off-Label Prescribing of Drugs in Specialty Headache Practice" *Headache* 44.7 (2004): 636–641.

Loftus, Stephen. "Pain and Its Metaphors: A Dialogical Approach" *Journal of Medical Humanities* 32 (2011): 213–230.

Lollar, Donald J. and Rune J. Simeonsson. "Diagnosis to Function: Classification for Children and Youths" *Journal of Developmental and Behavioral Pediatrics* 26.4 (Aug. 2005): 323–330.

Low, Rodolfo. *Victory over Migraine: The Breakthrough Study That Explains What Causes It and How It Can be Completely Prevented*. New York: Henry Holt & Co., 1987.

Mack, Jennifer W. and Joanne Wolfe. "Early Integration of Pediatric Palliative Care: For Some Children, Palliative Care Starts at Diagnosis" *Current Opinion in Pediatrics* 18 (2006): 10–14.

Macpherson, C. "Undertreating Pain Violates Ethical Principles" *Journal of Medical Ethics* 35.10 (2009): 603–606.

Margetts, Edward L. "Trepanation of the Skull by the Medicine-Men of Primitive Cultures, with Particular Reference to Present-Day Native East African Practice" in *Diseases in Antiquity: A Survey of the Diseases, Injuries, and Surgery of Early Populations*. Eds. Don Brothwell and A. T. Sandison. Springfield, IL: Charles C. Thomas, 1967: 673–701.

Marko, Georg. "My Painful Self; Health Identity Construction in Discussion Forums on Headaches and Migraine" *AAA: Arveiten aus Anglistik und Amerikanistik* 37.2 (2012): 245–272.

Marston, Joan. "Why Should Children Suffer? Children's Palliative Care and Pain Management" in *Children of the Drug War: Perspectives on the Impact of Drug Policies on Young People*. Ed. Damon Barrett. New York: International Debate Education Association, 2011: 219–236.

Martin, Graham. "Why Trepan? Contributions from Medical History and the South Pacific" in *Trepanation: History, Discovery, Theory*. Eds. Robert Arnott, Stanley Finger, and C. U. M. Smith. Lisse, Netherlands: Swets and Zeitlinger, 2003: 323–345.

Martinovic, Michelle. Personal Interview. 20 March, 2015.

Mateen, Farrah J., Joseph P. Geer, Kevin Frick, and Marco Carone. "Neurologic Disorders in Medicaid vs. Privately Insured Children and Working-Age Adults" *Neurology: Clinic Practice* 4.2 (Apr. 2014): 136–145.

Matheson, Whitney. "A Chat with. . .: Artist and 'H Day' Author Renee French" *USA Today*. 8 Nov. 2010. Web. 11 Aug. 2013.

Matossian, Mary Kilbourne. "Ergot and the Salem Witchcraft Affair" in *Witches of the Atlantic World: A Historical Reader and Primary Sourcebook*. Ed. Elaine G. Breslaw. New York: New York University Press, 2000: 467–479.

———. *Poisons of the Past: Molds, Epidemics, and History*. New Haven: Yale University Press, 1989.

Matthews, W. B. "Footballer's Migraine" *The British Medical Journal* 2.5809 (May 6, 1972): 326–327.

Mayes, Rick, Catherine Bagwell, and Jennifer Erkulwater. *Medicating Children: ADHD and Pediatric Mental Health*. Cambridge: Harvard University Press, 2009.

McAllister, William B. *Drug Diplomacy in the Twentieth Century: An International History*. New York: Routledge, 2000.

McDonagh, Patrick. *Idiocy: A Cultural History*. Liverpool: Liverpool University Press, 2008.

McElrath, Joseph R., Jesse S. Crisler, and Susan Shillinglaw, eds. *John Steinbeck: The Contemporary Reviews*. Cambridge: Cambridge University Press, 1996.

McEwan, Ian. *Atonement*. 2001. New York: Anchor Books, 2003.

McGrath, Patricia and Loretta M. Hillier. *The Child with Headache: Diagnosis and Treatment*. Seattle: International Association for the Study of Pain, 2001.

McGrath, Patrick J. and Kenneth D. Craig. "Developmental and Psychological Factors in Children's Pain" *The Pediatric Clinics of North America* 36.4 (1989): 823–826.

McGrath, Patrick J. and Anita M. Unruh. "The Social Context of Neonate Pain" *Clinical Perinatology* 29 (2002): 555–572.

McHugh, Susan. *Animal Stories: Narrating Across Species Lines*. Minneapolis: University of Minnesota Press, 2011.

McKay, Jno B. "A Clinical History of Three Interesting Cases of Morphinism" *Denver Medical Times* 27 (1907): 463–468.

McRuer, Robert. *Crip Theory: Cultural Signs of Queerness and Disability*. New York: New York University Press, 2006.

McTavish, Jan R. *Pain and Profits: The History of the Headache and Its Remedies in America*. New Brunswick: Rutgers University Press, 2004.

Meehan, William P. *Kids, Sports, and Concussion: A Guide for Coaches and Parents*. New York: Praeger, 2011.

Meier, Deborah. *In Schools We Trust: Creating Communities of Learning in an Era of Testing and Standardization*. Boston: Beacon Press, 2002.

Melville, Herman. *Moby-Dick, or the Whale*. 1851. New York: Random House, 1930.

Merikangas, Kathleen R., D. E. Stevens, and J. Angst. "Headache and Personality: Results of a Community Sample of Young Adults" *Journal of Psychiatric Research* 27.2 (1993): 187–196.

Metsähonkala, Liisa. "Social Environment and Headache in 8–9-Year-Old Children: A Follow-Up Study" *Headache* 38 (1998): 222–228.

Meunchen, Ashley. Telephone Interview. 22 October, 2015.

"Migraine May Cause Death" *The Science News-Letter* 78.14 (Oct. 1, 1960): 221.

Miller, Alice. *The Body Never Lies*. New York: W. W. Norton, 2006.

———. *The Untouched Key: Tracing Childhood Trauma in Creativity and Destructiveness*. 1988. Trans. Hildegarde Hannum and Hunter Hannum. New York: Anchor/Doubleday, 1990.

Miller, Toby. "Panic Between the Lips in Moral Panics: Attention-Deficit Hyperactivity Disorder and Ritalin®" in *Moral Panics over Contemporary Children and Youth*. Ed. Charles Krinsky. Farnham: Ashgate Publishing, 2008: 143–165.

Minot, G. R. "The Role of a Low Carbohydrate Diet in the Treatment of Migraine Headache" *The Medical Clinics of North America* 7 (1923): 715–728.

Mintz, Susannah B. *Hurt and Pain: Literature and the Suffering Body*. New York: Bloomsbury, 2014.

———. "On a Scale from 1 to 10: Life Writing and Lyrical Pain" *Journal of Literary and Cultural Disability Studies* 5.3 (2011): 243–260.

Mitchell, David T. and Sharon L. Snyder. *The Biopolitics of Disability: Neoliberalism, Ablenationalism, and Peripheral Embodiment*. Ann Arbor: University of Michigan Press, 2015.

———. *Narrative Prosthesis: Disability and the Dependencies of Discourse*. Ann Arbor: University of Michigan Press, 2000.

Morris, A. M. "Footballer's Migraine" *The British Medical Journal* 2.5816 (Jun. 24, 1972): 769–770.

Morris, David. *The Culture of Pain*. Berkeley: University Cal Press, 1991.

Morrison, Grant. "The Coyote Gospel" Illus. by Chas Truog and Doug Hazelwood. *Animal Man* 5 (1988).

Mullins, C. Daniel, Prasun R. Subedi, Paul J. Healey, and Robert J. Sanchez. "Economic Analysis of Triptan Therapy for Acute Migraine: A Medicaid Perspective" *Pharmacotherapy* 27.8 (2007): 1092–1101.

Munro, Joyce Underwood. "The Invisible Made Visible: The Fairy Changeling as a Folk Articulation of Failure to Thrive in Infants and Children" in *The Good People: New Fairylore Essays*. Ed. Peter Narváez. Lexington: University of Kentucky Press, 1991: 251–283.

Murison, Justine S. "The Paradise of Non-Experts: The Neuroscientific Turn of the 1840s United States" in *The Neuroscientific Turn: Transdisciplinarity in the Age of the Brain.* Eds. Melissa M. Littlefield and Jenell M. Johnson. Ann Arbor: University of Michigan Press, 2012: 29–48.

Murray, Stuart. *Representing Autism: Culture, Narrative, Fascination.* Liverpool: Liverpool University Press, 2008.

Murray, T. J. "The Neurology of Alice in Wonderland" *The Canadian Journal of Neurological Sciences* 9 (1982): 453–457.

Myers, Bernard. "A British Medical Association Lecture on the Nervous Child as Seen in Medical Practice" *The British Medical Journal* 2.3369 (Jul. 25, 1925): 158–162.

NBC Sports. "RotoWorld" Oct. 26, 2014. www.rotoworld.com/player/nfl/3698/player?r=1. Downloaded Oct. 27, 2014.

Neal, Helen. *The Politics of Pain.* New York: McGraw-Hill, 1978.

Nichols, Sharon Lynn. *Collateral Damage: How High-Stakes Testing Corrupts America's Schools.* Cambridge: Harvard Education Press, 2007.

Nietzsche, Friedrich. "Fate and History: Thoughts" 1862. in *The Nietzsche Reader.* Eds. Keith Ansell Pearson and Duncan Large. Malden, MA: Blackwell Publishing, 2006: 12–17.

———. "Four Letters (1888–9)" in *The Nietzsche Reader.* Eds. Keith Ansell Pearson and Duncan Large. Malden, MA: Blackwell Publishing, 2006: 516–523.

———. *The Gay Science.* 1887. Trans. Walter Kaufmann, New York: Random House Vintage, 1974.

Noonan, John T. "The Experience of Pain by the Unborn" in *New Perspectives in Human Abortion.* Eds. Thomas W Hilgers, Dennis J Horan, and David Mall. Frederick, MO: University Publications of America, 1981.

Nutkiewicz, Michael. "Diagnosis versus Dialogue: Oral Testimony and the Study of Pediatric Pain" *Oral History Review* 35.1 (2008): 11–21.

O'Brien, Ruth. *Bodies in Revolt: Gender, Disability, and a Workplace Ethic of Care.* New York: Routledge, 2005.

O'Malley, Andrew. *The Making of the Modern Child: Children's Literature and Childhood in the Late Eighteenth Century.* New York: Routledge, 2003.

Opie, Iona and Peter Opie. *Children's Games in Street and Playground.* Oxford: Clarendon Press, 1969.

Orbán, Katalin. "Trauma and Visuality: Art Spiegelman's Maus and In the Shadow of No Towers" *Representations* 97.1 (2007): 57–89.

O'Shea, Tim. "Talking Comics with Tim" 11 Oct. 2010. Web. 18 Aug. 2013.

Oswald, Lori Jo. "Heroes and Victims: The Stereotyping of Animal Characters in Children's Realistic Animal Fiction" *Children's Literature in Education* 26.2 (1995): 135–149.

Palacio, R. J. *Wonder.* New York: Alfred A. Knopf, 2012.

Parini, Jay. *John Steinbeck: A Biography.* New York: Henry Holt, 1995.

Parra Diaz, Camila. Personal Interview. 19 May, 2011.

Passchier, J. and J. F. Orlebeke. "Headaches and Stress in Schoolchildren: An Epidemiological Study" *Cephalalgia* 5 (1985): 167–176.

Patsavas, Alyson. "Recovering a Cripistemology of Pain: Leaky Bodies, Connective Tissue, and Feeling Discourse" *Journal of Literary and Cultural Disability Studies* 8.2 (2014): 203–218.

Pernick, Martin S. *A Calculus of Suffering: Pain, Professionalism, and Anesthesia in Nineteenth-Century America.* New York: Columbia University Press, 1985.

Perrucci, Alissa. "The Politics of Fetal Pain" in *Abortion Under Attack.* Ed. Krista Jacob. Emeryville, CA: Seal Press, 2006: 137–142.

Petchesky, Rosalind Pollack. "Fetal Images: The Power of Visual Culture in the Politics of Reproduction" *Feminist Studies* 13.2 (Summer 1987): 263–292.

Podoll, Klaus. 13 August 2013. Email.

———. 23 August 2013. Email.

———. "Migraine Aura as Artistic Inspiration" *British Medical Journal* 297 (Dec. 14–31, 1988): 1670–1672.

Podoll, Klaus and Derek Robinson. "Lewis Carroll's Migraine Experiences" *The Lancet* 353 (Apr. 17, 1999): 1366.

———. *Migraine Art: The Experience from Within.* Foreword by Oliver Sacks. Berkeley: North Atlantic Books, 2008.

Pogrebin, Letty Cottin. "Do Americans Hate Children?" *Ms.* 12 (Nov. 1983): 47–50, 126–127.

Porter, Eleanor H. *Pollyanna.* 1913. New York: Bantam Doubleday Dell, 1986.

"Potter's Scar Placement Conjures Up Fan Buzz" *Edmonton Journal.* 12 Jul. 2001. Web. 7 Feb. 2015.

Price, Margaret. *Mad at School: Rhetorics of Mental Disability and Academic Life.* Ann Arbor: University of Michigan Press, 2011.

Ramachandran, V. S. *The Tell-Tale Brain: A Neuroscientist's Quest for What Makes Us Human.* New York: W. W. Norton, 2011.

Rautman, Gretchen. *My Secret: Me and My Body's Pain.* Illus. by Kathleen Schmiedeskamp. Raleigh, NC: Lulu, 2009.

Reiss, Suzanna. *We Sell Drugs: The Alchemy of U.S. Empire.* Oakland: University of California Press, 2014.

Restak, Richard M. "Alice in Migraineland" *Headache* 46 (2006): 306–311.

Rich, Michael, Steven Lamola, Jason Gordon, and Richard Chalfen. "Video Intervention/ Prevention Assessment: A Patient-Centered Methodology for Understanding the Adolescent Illness Experience" *Journal of Adolescent Health* 27 (2000): 155–165.

Richardson, Jack and Jennifer Eisenhauer. "Dr. Phil, Medical Theaters, Freak Shows, and Talking Couches: The Talking Stage as Pedagogical Site" *Journal of Literary and Cultural Disability Studies* 8.1 (2014): 67–80.

Roberts, Teri. *Living Well with Migraine Disease.* New York: HarperCollins, 2005.

Rolak, Loren A. "Literary Neurologic Syndromes" *Archives of Neurology* 48 (1991): 649–651.

Ross, Dorothea M. and Sheila Ross. *Childhood Pain: Current Issues, Research, and Management.* Munich: Urban and Schwarzenberg, 1988.

———. "Childhood Pain: The School-Aged Child's Viewpoint" *Pain* 20 (1984): 179–191.

Roos, Michael E. "The Walrus and the Deacon: John Lennon's Debt to Lewis Carroll" *The Journal of Popular Culture* 18.1 (1984): 19–29.

Roth, Melissa. *The Left Hand: How the Left-Handed Have Survived and Thrived in a Right-Handed World.* New York: M. Evans and Company, 2005.

Rothenberg, Michael B. "Is There an Unconscious National Conspiracy against Children in the United States?" *Clinical Pediatrics* 19.1 (1980): 15–24.

Rovner, Sandy. "Headaches: Portraits of Pain" *The Washington Post.* 26 Sept. 1989: Z12.

Rowling, Jason. Telephone Interview. 5 June, 2014.

Rowling, J. K. *Harry Potter and the Sorcerer's Stone.* New York: Scholastic, 1997.

Rozen, T. D., J. W. Swanson, P. E. Stang, S. K. McDonnell, and W. A. Rocca. "Increasing Incidence of Medically Recognized Migraine Headache in a United States Population" *Neurology* 53 (1999): 1468–1473.

Ruhrah, J. *Pediatrics of the Past*. New York: Paul B. Hoeber, 1925.

Russell, Marquetta F. Personal Interview. 22 July, 2011.

Russo, Ethan. "Cannabis for Migraine Treatment: The Once and Future Prescription? An Historical and Scientific Review" *Pain* 76 (1998): 3–8.

Sabatello, Maya. "Children with Disabilities: A Critical Appraisal" *International Journal of Children's Rights* 21 (2013): 464–487.

Sacks, Oliver. *Migraine*. 1970. New York: Random House, 1992.

Saint Louis, Catherine. "F. D. A. Approval of OxyContin Use for Children Continues to Draw Scrutiny" *The New York Times*. 8 Oct. 2015. Web. 8 Oct. 2015.

Santoscoy, Gilbert. Personal Interview. 26 June, 2014.

Savage, Jeff. *Terrell Davis*. New York: Lerner Publications, 2000.

Sayce. R. U. "The Origins and Development of the Belief in Fairies" *Folklore* 45.2 (1934): 99–143.

Scarry, Elaine. "Among School Children: The Use of Body Damage to Express Pain" *Interfaces* 26 (2006): 11–36.

———. *The Body in Pain: The Making and Unmaking of the World*. Oxford: Oxford University Press, 1985.

———. "The Difficulty of Imagining Other Persons" in *The Handbook of Interethnic Conflict*. Ed. Eugene Weiner. New York: Continuum, 1998: 40–62.

———. "Pain and Embodiment in Culture" in *Pain and Its Transformations: The Interface of Biology*. Eds. Sarah Coakley and Kay Kaufman Shelemay. Cambridge: Harvard University Press, 2007: 64–66.

———. *Resisting Representation*. New York: Oxford University Press, 1994.

Schalk, Sami. "Metaphorically Speaking: Ableist Metaphors in Feminist Writing" *Disability Studies Quarterly* 33.4 (2013). Web. 30 Apr. 2015.

Schechter, Neil L. "The Undertreatment of Pain in Children; an Overview" *The Pediatric Clinics of North America* 36 (1989): 781–794.

Schechter, Neil L., D. A. Allen, and K. Hanson. "Status of Pediatric Pain Control" *Pediatrics* 77.1 (1986): 11–15.

Scheffel, Carl. "The Etiology of Fifty Cases of Drug Addictions" *Medical Record* 94 (1918): 853–854.

Schott, G. D. "Communicating the Experience of Pain: The Role of Analogy" *Pain* 108 (2004): 209–212.

Schwartz, Alan. "Thousands of Toddlers Are Medicated for ADHD, Report Finds, Raising Worries" *New York Times*. 16 May 2014. Web. 7 Jun. 2014.

Scott, Ruth. "It Hurts Red: A Preliminary Study of Children's Perception of Pain" *Perceptual and Motor Skills* 47 (1978): 787–791.

Scwartz, Carly. "Thousands of Families Demand Legal Medical Marijuana for Their Critically Ill Kids" *The Huffington Post*. 22 Apr. 2015. Web. 23 Dec. 2015.

Shakespeare, Tom. "Book Review of *An Anthropologist on Mars* by Oliver Sacks" *Disability and Society* 11.1 (1996): 137–142.

Shapiro, Deb. *Your Body Speaks Your Mind: Decoding the Emotional, Psychological, and Spiritual Messages That Underlie Illness*. Boulder: Sounds True, 2006.

Shapiro, Joseph P. "Tiny Tims, Supercrips, and the End of Pity" in *No Pity: People with Disabilities Forging a New Civil Rights Movement*. Ed. Joseph Shapiro. New York: Random House, 1993: 12–40.

Sheftell, Fred. "Role and Impact of Over-the-Counter Medications in the Management of Headache" *Neurologic Clinics* 15.1 (1997): 187–198.

Sheftell, Fred, T. J. Steiner, and H. Thomas. "Harry Potter and the Curse of the Headache" *Headache* 47 (2007): 911–916.

Sheridan, Mary S. *Pain in America*. Tuscaloosa, AL: University of Alabama Press, 1992.

Sherry, Mark. *If I Only Had a Brain: Deconstructing Brain Injury*. New York: Routledge, 2006.

———. "Reading Me/Me Reading Disability" *Prose Studies: History, Theory, Criticism* 27.1–2 (2005): 163–175.

Shifflett, C. M. *Migraine Brains and Bodies*. Berkeley: North Atlantic Books, 2011.

Shildrick, Margrit. "Re-Imagining Embodiment: Prostheses, Supplements and Boundaries" *Somatechnics* 3.2 (2013): 270–286.

Sick: The Life and Death of Bob Flanagan, Supermasochist. Dir. Kirby Dick. Santa Monica: Lionsgate Home Entertainment, 1997.

Siebers, Tobin. *Disability Theory*. Ann Arbor: University of Michigan Press, 2008.

———. "In the Name of Pain" in *Against Health: How Health Became the New Morality*. Eds. Jonathan M. Metzl and Anna Kirkland. New York: New York University Press, 2010: 183–194.

The Silences of the Palace. Dir. Moufida Tlatli. Amorces Diffusion Capiltol Entertainment, 1994.

Sillanpää, Matti. "Changes in the Prevalence of Migraine and Other Headaches During the First Seven School Years" *Headache* 23 (1983): 15–19.

Sillanpää, Matti and Pirjo Anttila. "Increasing Prevalence of Headache in 7-Year-Old Schoolchildren" *Headache* 36 (1996): 466–470.

Silverstein, Alvin and Virginia B. Silverstein. *Headaches: All about Them*. New York: Lippincott, 1984.

Slap-Shelton, Laura. "Migraine Headache" in *Children with Complex Medical Issues in Schools: Neuropsychological Descriptions and Interventions*. Ed. Christine L. Castillo. New York: Springer Publishing, 2008: 353–366.

Slater, Jenny. *Youth and Disability: A Challenge to Mr. Reasonable*. Burlington: Ashgate, 2015.

Sleeter, Christine. "Why Is There Learning Disabilities? A Critical Analysis of the Birth of the Field in Its Social Context" in *The Formation of School Subjects: The Struggle for Creating an American Institution*. Ed. Thomas S. Popkewitz. New York: Falmer Press, 1987: 210–237.

Small, David. *Stitches: A Memoir*. New York: Norton, 2009.

Sontag, Susan. *Illness as a Metaphor and AIDS and Its Metaphors*. New York: Farrar, Strauss, and Giroux, 1977/1989.

Speer, Nathan. Personal Interview. 27 April, 2011.

Spronk, Sarah. "Realizing Children's Right to Health" *International Journal of Children's Rights* 22 (2014): 189–204.

Spurgeon, Tom. "CR Sunday Interview: Renée French" *The Comics Reporter*. 7 Jun. 2011. Web. 18 Aug. 2013.

Squier, Susan M. "So Long as They Grow Out of It: Comics, the Discourse of Developmental Normalcy, and Disability" *Journal of Medical Humanities* 29 (2008): 71–88.

Stafstrom, Carl E., S. R. Goldenholz, and D. A. Dulli. "Serial Headache Drawings by Children with Migraine: Correlation with Clinical Headache Status" *Journal of Child Neurology* 20.10 (2005): 809–813.

———. "The Usefulness of Children's Drawings in the Diagnosis of Headache" *Pediatrics* 109 (2002): 460–472.

Stang, P. E., P. A. Yanagihara, J. W. Swanson, C. M. Beard, W. M. O'Fallon, H. A. Guess, and L. J. Melton. "Incidence of Migraine Headache: A Population-Based Study in Olmsted County, Minnesota" *Neurology* 42.9 (Sept. 1992): 1657–1662.

Starfield, Barbara. "U.S. Child Health Worse Than Other Industrialized Countries" Sept. 16, 2004. www.jhsph.edu/news/news-releases/2004/starfield-child-health.html. Web. 6 Jul. 2014.

Stein, Ragnar. "Neurology in the Nordic Sagas" in *Neurology of the Arts*. Ed. Clifford Rose. London: Imperial College Press, 2004: 389–400.

Steinbeck, John. *The Wayward Bus*. 1947. New York: Penguin, 2006.

Stewart, Walter F., R. B. Lipton, D. D. Celentano, and M. L. Reed. "Prevalence of Migraine Headache in the United States: Relation to Age, Income, Race, and Other Sociodemographic Factors" *JAMA* 267.1 (Jan. 1, 1992): 64–69.

Stirling, Jeannette. *Representing Epilepsy: Myth and Matter*. Liverpool: Liverpool University Press, 2010.

Stratford, Karen Ray. *A Comparison of Nursing Service Demand in Title 1 Schools and Non-Title 1 Schools*. University of Nevada, Las Vegas. Thesis. 2013.

Tabachnick, Stephen E. "Autobiography as Discovery in *Epileptic*" in *Graphic Subjects: Critical Essays on Autobiography and Graphic Novels*. Ed. Michael Chaney. Madison: University of Wisconsin Press, 2011: 101–116.

Tan, Shaun. *The Arrival*. New York: Scholastic, 2006.

Tansey, E. M. "Ergot to Ergometrine: An Obstetric Renaissance?" in *Women and Modern Medicine*. Eds. Lawrence Conrad and Anne Hardy. Amsterdam: Editions Rodopi, 2011: 195–215.

Taussig, Michael T. "Reification and the Consciousness of the Patient" *Social Science of Medicine* 14B (1980): 3–13.

Tfelt-Hansen, Peer C. and Peter Koehler, "One Hundred Years of Migraine Research: Major Clinical and Scientific Observations from 1910 to 2010" *Headache* 51 (2011): 752–778.

That Beautiful Somewhere. Dir. Robert Budreau. Perf. Roy Dupuis and Jane McGregor. Loon Films, 2006. DVD.

Thernstrom, Melanie. *The Pain Chronicles: Cures, Myths, Mysteries, Prayers, Diaries, Brain Scans, Healing, and the Science of Suffering*. New York: Farrar, Straus and Giroux, 2010.

Theroux, Alexander. *The Primary Colors*. New York: Henry Holt, 1994: 159.

Thomas, G. N. W. "Sugar and Migraine" *The British Medical Journal* 2.3326 (Sept. 27, 1924): 598.

Thompson, Suzanne C. "Will It Hurt Less if I Can Control It? A Complex Answer to a Simple Question" *Psychological Bulletin* 90.1 (1981): 89–101.

Tietjen, Gretchen, J. L. Brandes, B. L. Peterlin, A. Eloff, R. M. Dafer, M. R. Stein, E. Drexler, V. T. Martin, S. Hutchinson, S. K. Aurora, A. Recober, N. A. Herial, C. Utley, L. White, and S. A. Khuder. "Childhood Maltreatment and Migraine (Parts I–II)" *Headache* 50.1 (Jan. 2010): 20–41.

Torres, Justin. *We the Animals*. New York: Houghton Mifflin, 2011.

Tuchman, Gaye. "Invisible Difference: On the Management of Children in Postindustrial Society" *Sociological Forum* 11.1 (Mar. 1996): 3–23.

van Vugt, Peter. "C. L. Dodgson's Migraine and Lewis Carroll's Literary Inspiration: A Neurolinguistic Perspective" *Linguistica Antverpiensia* 28 (1994) 151–161.

Vegni, E., E. Mauri, and E. A. Moja. "Stories from Doctors of Patients with Pain: A Qualitative Research on the Physicians Perspective" *Supportive Care in Cancer* 13 (2005): 18–25.

Vertosick, Frank T., Jr. *Why We Hurt: The Natural History of Pain*. New York: Harcourt, 2000.

Vickers, Margaret H. "Life at Work with 'Invisible' Chronic Illness (ICI): A Passage of Trauma – Turbulent, Random, Poignant" *Administrative Theory and Praxis* 20.2 (1998): 196–210.

Vidali, Amy. "Seeing What We Know: Disability and Theories of Metaphor" *Journal of Literary and Cultural Disability Studies* 4.1 (2010): 33–54.

Wailoo, Keith. *Pain: A Political History*. Baltimore: Johns Hopkins University Press, 2014.

Walco, Gary A., Robert C. Cassidy, and Neil L. Schechter. "The Ethics of Pain Control in Infants and Children" in *Pain in Infants, Children, and Adolescents*. Eds. Neil Schechter, Charles Berde. Philadelphia: Lippincott, Williams, and Wilkins, 2003: 157–168.

———. "Sounding Board: Pain, Hurt, and Harm – the Ethics of Pain Control in Infants and Children" *New England Journal of Medicine* 331.8 (1994): 541–544.

Warner, Judith. *We've Got Issues: Children and Parents in the Age of Medication*. New York: Penguin Books, 2010.

Webb, E. "Discrimination against Children" *Archives of Disease in Childhood* 89 (2004): 804–808.

Weiss, Bernard. "Synthetic Food Colors and Neurobehavioral Hazards: The View from Environmental Health Research" *Environmental Health Perspectives* 120.1 (2012): 1–5.

Wendell, Susan. "Unhealthy Disabled: Treating Chronic Illnesses as Disabilities" *Hypatia* 16.4 (2001): 17–33.

West, Paul. "The Lightning-Rod Man: The Migraine Headache as Heuristic Tool" *The Journal of General Education* 26.4 (Winter 1975): 291–300.

Wheeler, Elizabeth A. "No Monsters in This Fairy Tale: *Wonder* and the New Children's Literature" *Children's Literature Association Quarterly* 38.3 (Fall 2013): 335–350.

White, E. B. *The Annotated Charlotte's Web*. 1952. Illus. by Garth Williams. Ed. Peter F. Neumeyer. New York: HarperCollins, 1994.

Wilkins, A. J., J. Huang, and Y. Cao. "Prevention of Visual Stress and Migraine with Precision Spectral Filters" *Drug Development Research* 68.7 (2007): 469–475.

Wilkins, A. J., R. Patel, P. Adjamian, and B. J. W. Evans. "Tinted Spectacles and Visually Sensitive Migraine" *Cephalalgia* 22.9 (2002): 711–719.

Wilkinson, C. F., Jr. "Recurrent Migrainoid Headaches Associated with Spontaneous Hypoglycemia" *The American Journal of the Medical Sciences* 218 (1949): 209–212.

Williams, Ian and M. K. Czerwiec, eds. *Graphic Medicine Manifesto*. University Park: Pennsylvania State University Press, 2015.

Wilper, Andrew, Steffie Woolhandler, David Himmelstein, and Rachel Nardin. "Impact of Insurance Status on Migraine Care in the United States: A Population-Based Study" *Neurology* 74 (Apr. 2010): 1178–1183.

Wilson, James and Cynthia Lewiecki-Wilson. *Embodied Rhetorics: Disability in Language and Culture*. Carbondale: Southern Illinois University Press, 2001.

Winderman, Ira. "Hawks, Wade Migraine Too Much for Heat to Overcome in 98–92 Loss" *South Florida Sun Sentinel*. 4 Nov. 2015. Web. 4 Nov. 2015.

Winner, Paul and A. David Rothner. *Headache in Children and Adolescents*. Hamilton, Ontario: BC Decker, Inc., 2001.

Wojaczynska-Stanek, Katarzyna, R. Koprowski, Z. Wróbel, and M. Gola. "Headache in Children's Drawings" *Journal of Child Neurology* 23 (2008): 184–191.

Woodhouse, Barbara Bennett. *Hidden in Plain Sight: The Tragedy of Children's Rights from Ben Franklin to Lionel Tate*. Princeton: Princeton University Press, 2008.

Woods, Roger P., Marco Iacoboni, and John C. Mazziotta. "Brief Report: Bilateral Spreading Cerebral Hypoferfusion During Spontaneous Migraine Headache" *New England Journal of Medicine* 331.25 (1994): 1689–1692.

Woolf, Virginia. "On Being Ill" 1926. in *Collected Essays*. Ed. Leonard Woolf. New York: Harcourt, 1967: 317–329.

World Health Organization. *Weekly Epidemiological Record* 66 (1991): 321–328.

Yao, Lynne. "FDA Takes Step to Encourage Pediatric Drug Studies" *FDA Voice*. 26 Aug., 2013. Web. 6 Oct. 2013.

Zayas, V., F. Mainardi, F. Maggioni, and G. Zanchin. "Sympathy for Pontius Pilate: Hemicrania in M. A. Bulgakov's the Master and Margarita" *Cephalalgia* 27 (2006): 63–67.

Zelizer, Viviana. *Pricing the Priceless Child: The Changing Social Value of Children*. New York: Basic Books, 1985.

Zeller, Kane. Personal Interview. 17 April, 2011.

Zeltzer, Lonnie K. and Christina Blackelt Schlack. *Conquering Your Child's Chronic Pain: A Pediatrician's Guide for Reclaiming a Normal Childhood*. New York: HarperCollins, 2005.

Zernike, Kate and Melody Petersen. "Schools' Backing of Behavior Drugs Comes Under Fire" *New York Times*. Aug. 19, 2001. Downloaded May 23, 2014.

Index